Right Down Your Alley

The Complete Book of Bowling

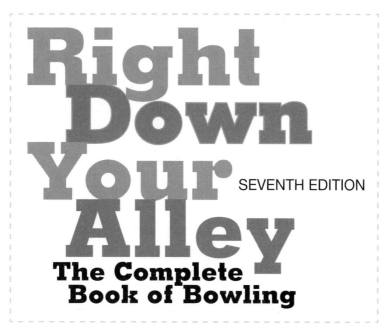

Right Down Your Alley

SEVENTH EDITION

The Complete Book of Bowling

Vesma Grinfelds

USBC and WPBA Hall of Fame Member

Bonnie Hultstrand

Professor Emeritus, Physical Education
University of Idaho

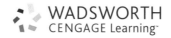

WADSWORTH
CENGAGE Learning

Australia • Brazil • Japan • Korea • Mexico • Singapore • Spain • United Kingdom • United States

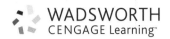

Right Down Your Alley: The Complete Book of Bowling, Seventh Edition

Vesma Grinfelds, Bonnie Hultstrand

Publisher/Executive Editor: Yolanda Cossio

Print Buyer: Judy Inouye

Right Acquisition Director: Bob Kauser

Permissions Editors: Dean Dauphinais (text & Image)

Production Manager: Matt Ballantyne

Acquisitions Editor: Laura Pople

Assistant Editor: Samantha Arvin

Developmental Editor: Liana Monari Sarkisian

Editorial Assistant/Associate: Kristina Chiapella

Technology Project Manager: Miriam Myers

Marketing Manager: Laura McGinn

Marketing Assistant/Associate: Elizabeth Wong

Art Director: John Walker

Production Service: PreMediaGlobal

Compositor: PreMediaGlobal

Manufacturing Manager: Marcia Locke

Cover Design: Betsy Bush

Cover Images: Masterfile

For product information and technology assistance, contact us at **Cengage Learning Customer & Sales Support, 1-800-354-9706**

For permission to use material from this text or product, submit all requests online at **cengage.com/permissions**
Further permissions questions can be emailed to **permissionrequest@cengage.com**

Library of Congress Control Number: 2010935920

ISBN-13: 978-0-8400-4807-3

ISBN-10: 0-8400-4807-6

Wadsworth
10 Davis Drive
Belmont, CA 94002-3098
USA

Cengage Learning is a leading provider of customized learning solutions with office locations around the globe, including Singapore, the United Kingdom, Australia, Mexico, Brazil, and Japan. Locate your local office at: **international.cengage.com/region**

Cengage Learning products are represented in Canada by Nelson Education, Ltd.

For your course and learning solutions, visit **academic.cengage.com**

Purchase any of our products at your local college store or at our preferred online store **www.cengagebrain.com**

Printed in the United States of America
1 2 3 4 5 6 7 14 13 12 11 10

Contents

A Historical Introduction to Bowling

Bowling might very well be the oldest form of recreation in the world today. An ancient version of a ball and pins resembling the current day bowling equipment was found in an Egyptian child's grave dating back to approximately 5200 BC. More than likely, Stone Age man may have enjoyed rolling rocks at other rocks. We know the ancient Polynesians played a game resembling bowling in which they used pins and balls made of stone and rolled the balls a distance similar to the length of the present lane bed.

It has also been recorded that about the time of Christ, rolling rocks down hills was a form of war maneuver used to bowl the enemy over with a strike. This skill was practiced by the soldiers in order to develop accuracy, and before long they found it to be a form of play. The Italian game of *bocce* (which is still widely played among persons of Italian descent) probably originated from this early war game.

The modern form of bowling at pins probably originated in the third century AD in ancient Germany, not as a sport but as a religious ceremony. German peasants during this time carried a *kegel*, a club used for protection. It became customary to take the *kegel* to church as a test of faith. The parishioner would bring his *kegel* and place it at the end of a cloister in the cathedral. He was then given a round stone to roll at the *kegel* which represented *heide*, the heathen. If the parishioner was successful in knocking down the *kegel*, he was said to have cleansed himself of sin. According to a nineteenth-century German historian, Wilhelm Pehle, this religious ceremony had its origin as early as the third or fourth century, and lasted less than two centuries.

As time passed, the game of bowling evolved into a recreational pastime rather than a religious ceremony. Martin Luther is said to have enjoyed the game of bowling and built a bowling lane for the younger members of his family. He is also credited with establishing the first set of rules for ninepin bowling. In ninepin, the pins were set in a diamond shape with the kingpin in the middle. The object was to knock down as many pins as possible without spilling the kingpin.

The game of bowling spread into the countries surrounding Germany. Austria, Spain, and Switzerland all adopted (and adapted) the game of bowling that usually was associated with inns and taverns into inside lanes made of sun-baked clay and wood. Around the same time, the Dutch in New Amsterdam established the game of ninepins (1650 AD), with the pins in a diamond pattern, and used an "alley" about a foot and a half wide and up to 99 feet long.

England also participated in bowling games as early as the fourteenth century, and by the year 1465, King Edward IV passed an edict forbidding "bowling-like" sports due to excessive gambling and the fact that he could not keep his troops focused on archery practice. The English then adapted the game to be played with a fingerless ball which was rolled on the lawn—the start of the game of lawn bowling, still in vogue in many settings today.

As the immigrants from these countries arrived in America, each brought with them their form of bowling. The game of ninepins was the form of bowling which was brought to America by the Dutch early in the seventeenth century. One of the early playing areas was in lower Manhattan, the spot still known as Bowling Green.

The game of bowling flourished in America and spread throughout the states. By the mid 1830s, it became a gambling sport which led to legislation banning ninepins in the 1840s. In order to circumvent the legislation, a tenth pin was added and all of the pins were placed in an equilateral triangle.

The new tenpin game did suffer in some areas from gambling but the biggest hindrance was the lack of uniform rules and equipment specifications. In 1895, the American Bowling Congress (ABC) was organized to standardize the playing rules and regulations. By the early 1900s, women became very interested in the game of bowling and formed their own organization to standardize the rules and sponsor competition. The Women's National Bowling Association, better known as the Women's International Bowling Congress (WIBC), was formed in 1916.

The interest for women in the game of bowling was heightened in 1927 when a local bowler, Mrs. Floretta McCutcheon, challenged and beat the world champion, Jimmy Smith, in an exhibition match. This match paved the way for the founding of the Mrs. McCutcheon School for Bowling. She influenced the growth of bowling through 1939 by giving thousands of clinics, lessons, and exhibitions throughout the nation. Another stabilizing influence came in 1932 with the formation of the Bowling Proprietors Association of America (BPAA). This organization was designed to improve the management of the sport and to stimulate the growth of bowling throughout the country through promotion programs and tournament sponsorship.

During World War II, bowling became a widespread recreational sport. It was one of the leisure activities provided by the armed forces for the many soldiers in training as well as for wounded veterans. In 1943, the National Bowling Council (NBC) was formed to coordinate all phases of bowling in the war effort. After the war, the NBC became an informational clearing house and legislative liaison organization for the sport. For many years, the NBC served as national coordinator for the sport of bowling. Bowling has been recognized throughout the world and in 1988, South Korea had it as an exhibition sport in the Olympic Games held there.

Bowling attracts millions of participants. With the addition of new, attractive bowling centers with automatic pinsetting and scoring machines, bowling has become a family sport. By 1970, the nation's most popular indoor participation sport was being enjoyed by nearly 52 million Americans of all ages. As of today, approximately 60 million people in the U.S. go bowling at least once a year and about 7 million of them compete in sanctioned league play.

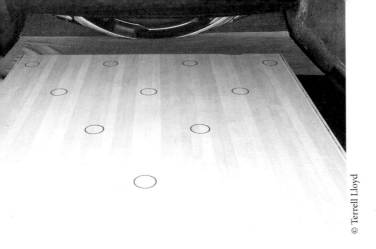

1

Understanding the Basics

On the surface, the game of bowling appears quite simple. The bowler takes an approach, rolls a fairly heavy ball down a 60-foot lane, and with two attempts tries to knock down the ten pins placed in a triangular fashion at the end of the lane. However, as the bowler delves into the mechanics of bowling, he or she finds a much more complicated game. We hope that in the next few chapters of this text the mysteries of successful bowling will be uncovered so each person may find that measure of success and knowledge that are sought. It is true that each bowler establishes his or her own style. However, truly successful bowlers seem to have many attributes in common: (1) They all have a smooth, flowing approach and delivery; (2) they all have excellent timing, balance, and flexibility during the approach and delivery; (3) their swing and approach is absolutely consistent on each delivery; (4) they have complete concentration, poise, and confidence; and (5) each has developed a system of adjustment to assist in compensating for outside forces where bowlers have little control, such as varying lane conditions. The above attributes do not just happen. They are practiced, through and through, and then grooved to the extent of becoming automatic.

The key to success in bowling lies in knowing the game inside and out, and being able to groove the entire approach, swing, and delivery where consistency is an absolute.

In the following chapters, we intend to present all of the information necessary for a bowler to achieve his or her potential. The material presented has been tried and proven by the best in the world.

Features of the Ball, Pins, and Lanes

Understanding ball, lane, and pin composition, and the dimensions of each, will aid the bowler in grasping the mechanical and mathematical concepts involved in bowling.

Bowling Ball

Bowling balls range from 8 to 16 pounds in weight and are constructed of hard rubber, synthetic plastic, urethane, or reactive resin materials. The number of finger holes in the ball varies from two to five, but the ball with three finger holes is the most common.

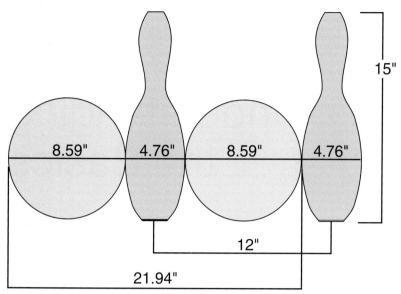

FIGURE 1.1 Relative dimensions of ball and pins.

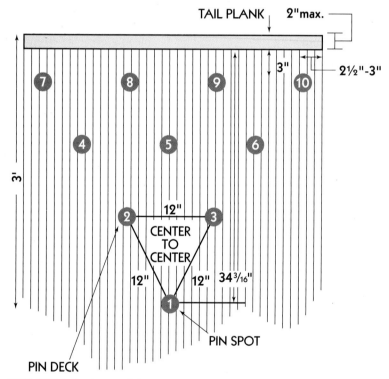

FIGURE 1.2 In an ABC regulation bowling lane, the pins are arranged in a 36-inch equilateral triangle. Each pin is 12 inches from the adjacent pin, center to center.

The finger holes in the bowling balls are drilled at different sizes, widths, and angles to fit the grip and size desired by the individual bowler (see Chapter 2). No matter what the weight, the ball measures approximately 27 inches in circumference and about 8½ inches in diameter (Figure 1.1).

Bowling Pins

Bowling pins are made of durable materials, usually hard rock maple covered by a thin plastic coating. Many bowling establishments are replacing these maple pins with synthetic pins that tend to last longer. These pins are 15 inches in height and 15 inches in circumference around the belly of the pin. The diameter is approximately 4¾ inches through the widest part (Figure 1.1). According to the United States Bowling Congress (USBC), pins may be no lighter than 3 pounds 6 ounces, and no heavier than 3 pounds 10 ounces. Furthermore, the set of pins in service at an establishment must all be of the same weight. On the bottom of the pin there is a nylon cap to protect it from wear and tear. Taking these specifications into consideration, it is interesting to note that a pin will topple when it moves 10 degrees off its vertical axis.

There are ten pins set on the lane in a 36-inch equilateral triangle, with each pin around the perimeter of the triangle and across the rows spread 12 inches apart, center to center (Figure 1.2).

Interesting Note: In examining the ball dimensions in relation to the pins, it is found that a single pin left standing could be contacted by the ball anywhere within a 22-inch area. It should also be noted that a ball cannot pass directly between two adjoining pins without contacting one or both of them (Figure 1.1).

The pins are numbered from front to back, always starting from left and going to the right. Before proceeding, the reader must memorize the pins by their correct number (Figure 1.3).

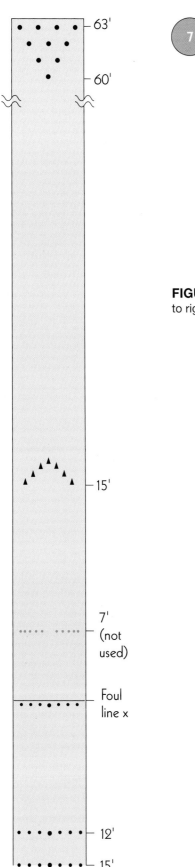

FIGURE 1.4   Relative distance of lane and approach markings from the foul line.

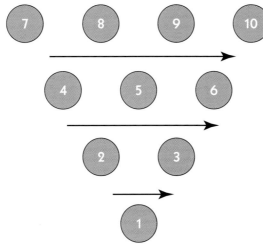

Pins on deck

FIGURE 1.3   The pins are numbered from left to right.

Lane Features and Dimensions

For a bowler to understand the bulk of material yet to be presented in this text, it is imperative to understand and be able to identify the different parts of the lane and its dimensions.

The bowling area is divided into four segments—the approach, the lane, the pin deck, and the pit area.

The Approach

The **approach** is the area found toward the back of the lane where bowlers take their steps and swing prior to the delivery of the ball. The approach is made up of laminated boards that are a little over an inch in width and about 4 inches thick set on end. These boards match the 39 boards that make up the lane in front of the approach area.

Usually on this approach, a bowler may identify three rows of dots extending parallel to the foul line. These dots are known as locator dots and are used by bowlers in finding their proper stance. The first row of locator dots can be found 2 to 3 inches behind the foul line. The other two rows are found 12 and 15 feet, respectively, from the

foul line (Figure 1.4). The dots are equally placed five boards apart and the center dot is in the center of the approach, which corresponds to the 20th board in the center of the lane.

The Lane

The **lane** is the area in front of the approach and foul line where the ball rolls to encounter the pins. The width of the lane is approximately 42 inches, made up of 39 laminated boards slightly over an inch in width plus a narrower filler board usually found somewhere between the edge board and first arrow on the left. The length of the lane from the foul line to the center of the head pin is 60 feet (Figure 1.4). In the traditional lanes, the first one-third of the lane, plus the outside board, and the area under the pins is constructed of hard maple that is extremely durable. The remainder of the lane to the head pin is constructed of pine. Because pine is much softer and contains more grain, it assists the bowling ball in "grabbing" the lane, resulting in greater hooking action. ***Note:*** There are also many synthetic lanes made of laminates that have a wood-like appearance. The dimensions and markings on these lanes are the same as on wood lanes.

Self Evaluation QUESTIONS ?

1. How many boards make up a bowling lane?
2. How many boards apart are the locator dots placed?
3. What is the minimum length of a bowling approach?

The Pin Deck and Pit Area

On the lane area, we find 7 large markings placed in an inverted V formation, known as **target arrows**.

These target arrows have special significance to each bowler, as they

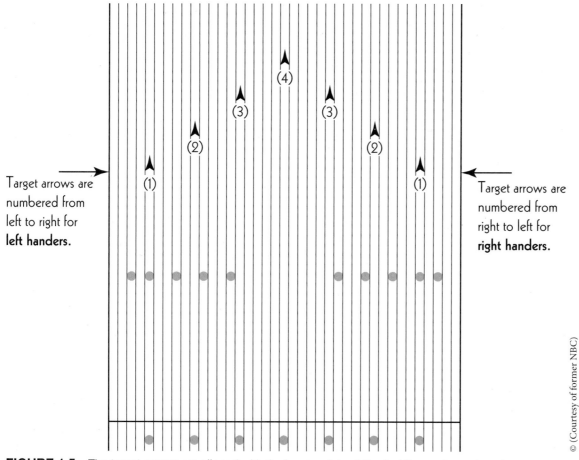

Target arrows are numbered from left to right for **left handers.**

Target arrows are numbered from right to left for **right handers.**

© (Courtesy of former NBC)

FIGURE 1.5   The target arrows are aligned with the locator dots at the foul line and are placed on every 5th board. **Note:** The spots between the foul line and target area *do not* line up with the target arrows and the locator dots. These spots are not used for our purposes.

Self Evaluation **QUESTIONS** ?

1. How many boards apart are the target arrows?
2. Are they in line with the locator dots on the approach?
3. How many boards make up the width of a lane?
4. How far is it from the foul line to the head pin?

help bowlers to focus on a specific target while delivering the ball, a procedure known as **spot bowling**. These target arrows are located 15 feet from the foul line with the center arrow on the 20th board. Just as on the approach, these arrows are also spaced five boards apart and are in perfect alignment (Figure 1.5). For right handers, this means that the third arrow from the right corresponds with the 15th board, the second arrow is on the 10th board, and

the first arrow is located on the 5th board (Figure 1.5).

Please Note: Left handers number these target arrows from left to right. For left handers, this means that the third arrow from the left corresponds to the 15th board, the second arrow from the left is on the 10th board, and the first arrow on the left is on the 5th board (Figure 1.5).

Halfway between the foul line and the target arrows, there is a row of dots called the spots. These spots are *not* lined up with the other locator dots or target arrows and are of little or no use to the average bowler. The spots are of value to higher average bowlers, those who are extremely nearsighted, or those who have physical handicaps.

The area of the lane where the pins are set is called the **pin deck** (Figure 1.6). It is approximately

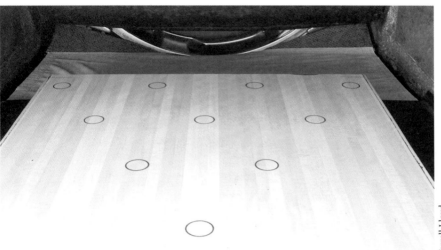

FIGURE 1.6   The markings on the pin deck denote where the pins will be placed.

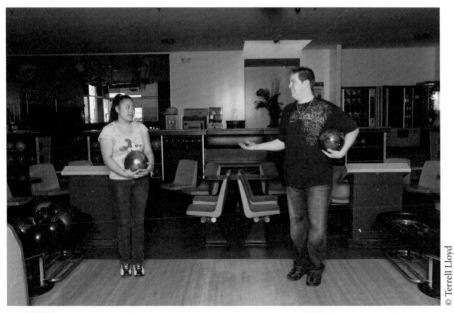

FIGURE 1.7   A bowler on the right takes his or her turn first.

area is recessed in order to catch the pins before they have a chance to bounce back out on the lane. It usually contains a moving belt that carries the ball back to the ball return and the pins into the automatic pinsetter.

Etiquette and Safety

There are many commonly accepted rules of **etiquette** that everyone should follow upon entering the bowling establishment. By using common sense and following these basic rules of etiquette, we will assist the management in keeping maintenance costs down, be respected and appreciated by others on the lanes, and help make the game of bowling pleasant and safe for all.

Basic Rules of Etiquette and Safety

- Before stepping onto the lane, check to make sure the bowlers on the adjoining lanes are not in their stance or taking their approach. The rule is: **Only one person on the approach at a time.** If you both step up on the approach at the same time, **yield to the person on the right** (Figure 1.7).
- Bowling is a sport that requires intense concentration. Therefore, refrain from disturbing any bowler in his or her approach. Loud noises and constant movement are very distracting to all.
- Restrict your body English and confine your elation or disappointment to your own lane or within yourself. Kicking the ball return or other equipment doesn't help anyone.
- After you have delivered the ball, walk straight back and step off the approach while waiting for the return of the ball (Figure 1.8).

36 inches in depth and is made of hardwood and durable synthetic materials to take the wear and tear of falling and flying pins.

To the sides of the pin deck are side partitions called **kickbacks** that help contain the pins and assist pin action on the pin deck. These kickbacks span the entire area from opposite the head pin to the rear cushion found above the pit area.

The **pit area** is approximately 4¾ inches below the surface of the pin deck and extends another 30 inches back to the cushion. This

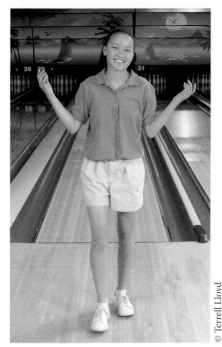

FIGURE 1.8   No matter how pleased you are with the result, confine your elation to your own lane and walk straight back from the foul line.

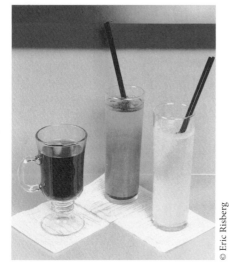

FIGURE 1.9   Food and drink should remain behind the settee area.

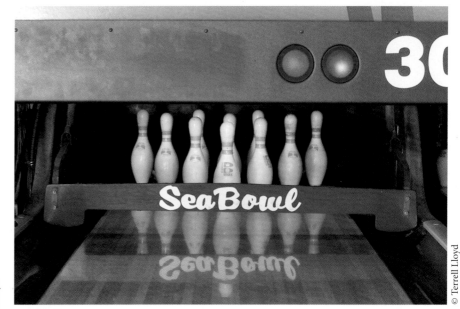

FIGURE 1.10   When the sweep is down in front of the pins, do *not* bowl.

- Take a *reasonable* amount of time while on the approach area but think of others. Many people become irritated if they have to wait too long for someone else.
- Use only *your* ball, towel, resin, and other equipment unless you have permission to borrow someone else's.
- Keep refreshments out of the bowler's settee area. Spilled liquids present problems to all bowlers (Figure 1.9).
- Be prepared to bowl when it is your turn. Plan your absences from the lane so no one will have to wait for you to return.
- Change into your bowling shoes before entering the bowling area. This will keep the area free from mud, water, and dirt that may be picked up by bowler's shoes and carried onto the lanes.
- Refrain from blaming someone else or equipment for your mistakes. More than likely it is your fault when things go wrong.
- Refrain from giving advice to others unless they ask for your help.
- Make sure the ball sweep is up before you deliver the ball (Figure 1.10).

- Avoid lofting the ball. This is damaging to the lanes as well as distracting to others (Figure 1.11).
- Avoid wearing long skirts, long floppy pants, floppy sleeves, or jewelry which may get tangled during the approach and cause a mishap.
- When lifting your bowling ball from the rack, to avoid pinched fingers and back strain, place both hands on the ball (one on each side), bend your knees, and lift by straightening the legs (Figure 1.12).
- Avoid going beyond the foul line (Figure 1.13).
- Respect the rights and privacy of others by *not* using your cell phone during bowling (Figure 1.14).

If you follow these simple rules, bowling will be more enjoyable to all. Remember the basic rule of good manners: **Be Considerate of Others**.

In a Nutshell:

- In order to become a good bowler you must groove the approach, the swing, and the delivery. This can only be accomplished through good practice.

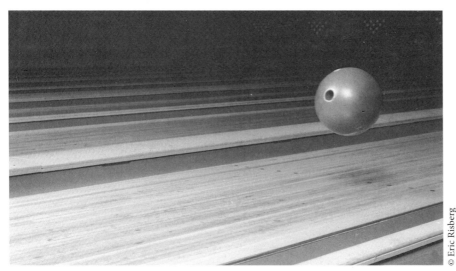

FIGURE 1.11 Do not loft the ball. This lofted delivery is 7 feet forward of the foul line and has not yet touched the lane.

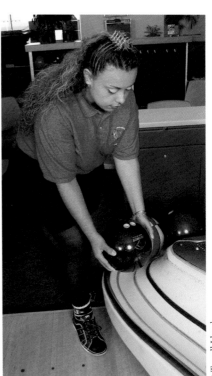

FIGURE 1.12 The proper way to remove a ball from the ball rack, minimizing the chances of hand or finger injury.

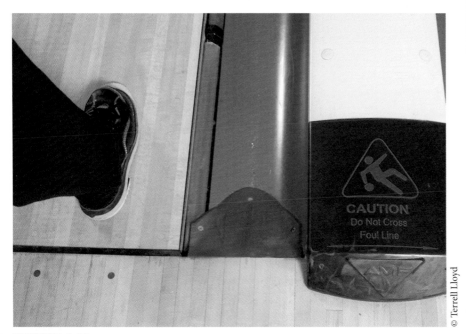

FIGURE 1.13 Do not step over the foul line.

- The bowling pins are set in a precise 36-inch equilateral triangle, are spaced 12 inches apart from center to center, and are numbered from left to right.
- The head pin is located on the 20th board and is 60 feet from the foul line.
- The approach is a minimum of 15 feet in length and has three sets of locator dots. These locator dots are used to assist the bowler in exact foot

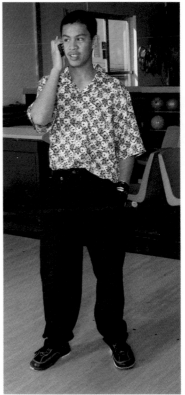

FIGURE 1.14 Respect the rights and privacy of others by *not* using your cell phone during bowling.

placements on his or her stance and approach.

- The locator dots are spaced five boards apart with the center dot on the 20th board. The dots and boards are always counted from the outside edge of the lane toward the center. For right handers, this is from right to left. For left handers, this is from left to right.

- The target arrows used for aiming in spot bowling are 15 feet in front of the foul line. They are also spaced five boards apart and are in direct line with the locator dots on the approach.

- Remember the basic rule of good manners: **Be Considerate of Others**.

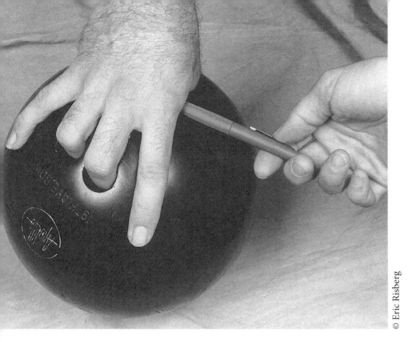
© Eric Risberg

2

Preparing for Action

Selection of Proper Equipment

Proper selection of equipment is essential for bowling success. Two basic equipment needs are (1) a pair of bowling shoes that are properly fitted and (2) a well-fitted ball.

Bowling Shoes

The **bowling shoes** rented at a bowling establishment are dual-purpose shoes that can be used by right or left handers because both the left and right soles are made of sliding material. When renting shoes, make sure that they fit comfortably and will slide at the end of the approach. Care must be taken when purchasing a pair of bowling shoes because they are made differently for left- and right-handed bowlers. The soles of most higher-quality shoes are constructed to give one foot some traction, while giving the other foot a sole for sliding purposes. **For right handers**, sliding at the foul line when delivering the ball is done on the left foot. In order to ensure a smooth slide, the left sole is usually made of leather. The right foot is used for traction so the right sole of the shoe is usually rubber with a leather tip.

For left handers, sliding at the foul line when delivering the ball is done on the right foot. Therefore, the right sole is usually made of leather to ensure a smooth slide. The left foot, used for traction, will use a shoe with a rubber sole with a leather tip (Figure 2.1).

Bowling Ball

To provide consistency, it is desirable for an individual to purchase a **bowling ball** and have it professionally selected and fitted. If this is not possible, then care must be exercised when selecting a "house" ball. It should be heavy enough to add stability to the swing, and yet not so heavy that it causes the shoulder to drop. Keep in mind, a heavier ball will have less deflection when it hits the pins, resulting in better pin coverage.

We recommend the following guidelines:

- For children under twelve, use a bowling ball that is 1 pound for every 10 pounds of body weight. This should come close to eight-year-olds using an 8-pound ball; a ten-year-old using a 10-pound ball, and so on.
- Most beginning women bowlers should be able to start with

FIGURE 2.1 Soles of bowling shoes are not all identical.

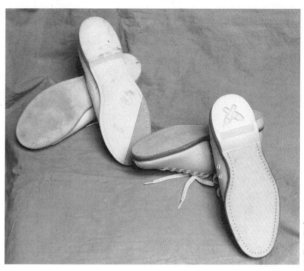

© Eric Risberg

an 11- or 12-pound ball, and as they progress they can move to a heavier ball.

● Most beginning male bowlers should be able to start with a 14- or 15-pound ball. Eventually, they may also want to move to a heavier ball.

After attending to the weight of the ball, the next consideration is hand and finger fit. The two most important factors to consider are the size of the thumb and finger holes and the span from the thumb to the fingers.

The thumb should comfortably and snugly fit into the thumb hole. It should come out of the hole with a little resistance but without popping. If the thumb hole is too large, many problems will arise from trying to grip the ball much too tightly with the thumb joint. A common error is "Knuckling" the ball. This is when the thumb in the hole bends so that the top of the thumb rubs against the hole. This is usually found when the thumb hole is too large or if the bowler is gripping the ball strongly. It should benefit that the finger should be pressing flat against the hole. The finger holes should fit the fingers fairly snugly and should allow the fingers to come out smoothly and without resistance.

The second important element in obtaining a proper fit is determining the span or distance between the thumb and the fingers according to the preferred grip—**conventional, fingertip,** or **semi-fingertip** (Figure 2.2).

The most common grip that has the shortest span is the **conventional grip**. Most "house" balls are drilled with this grip, which potentially allows the bowler to develop a high degree of accuracy and ball control. The second most popular grip with the largest span is the **fingertip grip**. It is used by consistent and highly skilled bowlers looking to achieve a higher degree of hook power and pin action. The **semi-fingertip** span is slightly wider than the conventional yet shorter than the fingertip, and is potentially useful for a bowler to increase the lift imparted at the point of release.

Most novice and intermediate bowlers use the conventional grip (Figure 2.3). In order to find the proper span for the **conventional grip**, place the thumb all the way into the thumb hole. Making sure that the wrist remains straight, extend the fingers across the span area of the ball. The lines on the second knuckle of your middle finger should exceed the edge of the finger hole closest to the thumb by about ¼ of an inch.

FIGURE 2.2
Different types of grips: Conventional; Fingertip; (c) Semi-fingertip.

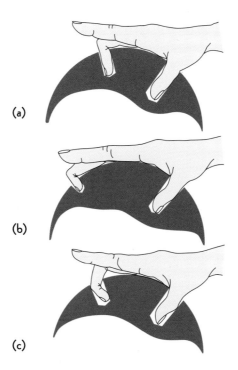

(a)

(b)

(c)

The second most popular bowling grip is the **fingertip**. Because the span is wider in this fingertip grip than in the conventional grip, measurement is made by using the first joint of the fingers instead of the second joint as in the conventional grip. To find the proper fit for the fingertip ball, place the thumb all the way into the thumb hole and extend the fingers over the surface of the ball. The line of the first joint will land right in the middle of the finger hole. If the ball fits correctly with the thumb and fingers in the ball, the second knuckle should be sticking up in the air slightly and forming a little triangle (Figure 2.4). If it is flat against the surface of the ball, the span is too long and the evidence will be burnt fingertips or excessive calluses. To ensure a properly drilled fingertip ball, a professional driller in a reputable pro shop should be sought.

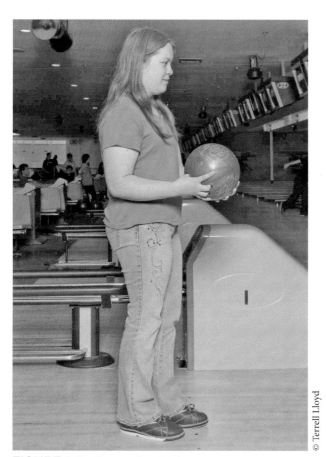

FIGURE 2.3 Conventional grip.

© Terrell Lloyd

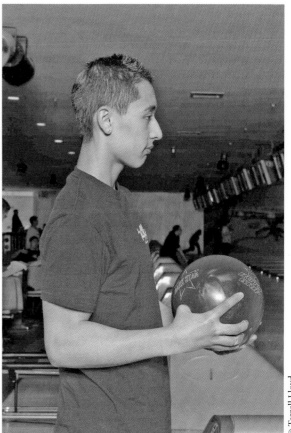

FIGURE 2.4 Fingertip grip.

© Terrell Lloyd

Conventional vs. Fingertip Discussion:

In comparing the advantages and disadvantages of the aforementioned conventional and fingertip grips, one finds that neither is perfect. Of the two, the conventional grip probably helps develop greater accuracy. The major disadvantage of the conventional grip is that the hooking action is only minimal because so much of the hand is inside the ball. The thumb comes out first, but, due to the compactness of the fingers, not enough time elapses for proper hand action to take place. This results in reduced hooking action with less pin carry.

The fingertip ball may be less accurate than the conventional grip but has a greater pin carry due to an increased hooking action. This greater hooking action is a result of greater lift and more revolutions that can be imparted on the ball with the wider span.

The third type of grip, the **semi-fingertip**, was designed to combine the advantages of both the conventional and fingertip—the control and accuracy of the conventional and the extra hooking action of the fingertip. The span is equidistant between the two first joints of the fingers. This particular grip has been found unsatisfactory primarily because the fingers cannot bend at the location between the two joints. This causes the fingers to grip the back of the hole and often causes discomfort to the bowler. It has not been as successful as originally anticipated and is not highly recommended.

Holding the Ball

To obtain maximum accuracy and consistency, it is absolutely essential that the hand position be held constant throughout the stance, swing,

Self Evaluation QUESTIONS?

1. What are two important considerations in properly fitting a bowling ball?
2. What are the three basic grips found in bowling balls?
3. How would you find the proper span for a conventional grip?

and delivery. This action will assist in allowing the ball to be delivered exactly the same on each ball delivery.

The most effective ball delivery is the one that results in the ball hooking slightly at the end of the ball roll into the strike pocket or proper selected key pin. This delivery is called a **hook ball** and is highly desirable, because there is an off-center ball rotation which allows the ball to enter the pins at a slight angle, minimizing deflection and maximizing "digging" action (Figure 2.5A and 2.5B).

This entire action, in turn, results in maximum **pin carry** by splattering the pins more sideways as the ball continues to roll into the 5 pin in the center of the triangle. The ball rotation imparted on the ball is merely an automatic result of the fingers applying upward pressure or lift on the ball from the 4 o'clock position by right handers and the 8 o'clock position for left handers, both being applied off the center of the ball.

Note: It is the authors' belief that due to the hook ball's superiority in pin action over the straight ball, all bowlers should learn from the very beginning the hook ball delivery. Therefore, all further discussion will be surrounding the roll of the hook ball and its effective use.

In finding the correct hand position for the **hook ball**, visualize the ball with a clock face on it. The

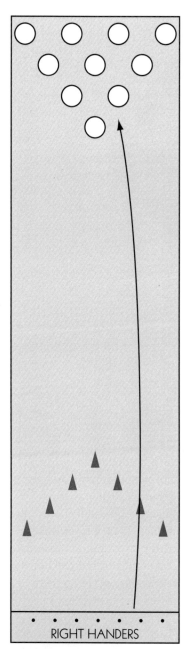

FIGURE 2.5A Right Handers—The path of a hook ball due to the fingers lifting off the center of the ball from the 4 o'clock position. The result is a counter-clockwise rotation.

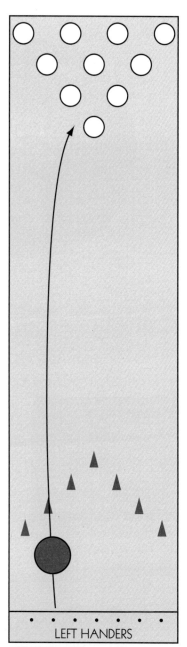

FIGURE 2.5B Left Handers—The path of a hook ball of a left hander where fingers lift off the center of the ball from the 8 o'clock position, resulting in a clockwise rotation.

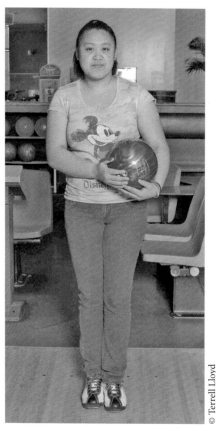

FIGURE 2.6 When taking the stance position, the ball is held in the non-bowling hand.

center of the clock face is between the finger and thumb holes of the ball. Standing in the appropriate position with the ball supported in the non-bowling hand (Figure 2.6), the right-handed bowler places the thumb and finger holes in a 10

and 4 o'clock position, respectively (Figure 2.7). The left-handed bowler places the thumb at 2 and fingers at 8 o'clock (Figure 2.8).

Turning the ball face now slightly to the side while maintaining the 10 and 4 o'clock (right handers) or the 2 and 8 o'clock (left handers) positions, the fingers and thumb are inserted and the wrist will be found firm and straight in relation to the bowler's forearm (Figures 2.7 and 2.8).

Note: Good control is associated with gripping the ball firmly. Spread the two outside fingers apart and press downward against the surface of the ball with the tips of the fingers. This will help keep the wrist firm to create maximum control at delivery.

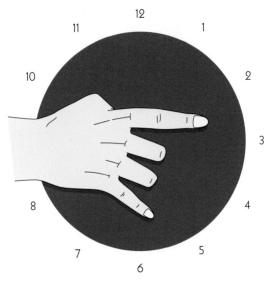

FIGURE 2.7   Right Handers—The 10–4 o'clock position used to deliver a hook ball.

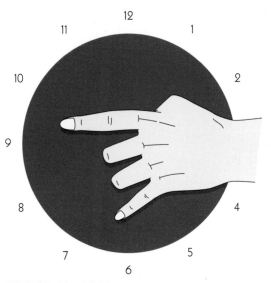

FIGURE 2.8   Left Handers—The 2–8 o'clock position used to deliver a hook ball.

Self Evaluation QUESTIONS?

1. Why is a hook ball recommended?
2. In what position are the thumb and fingers placed in the ball to roll a hook ball?
3. How can you firm the wrist while gripping the ball?

Aiming in Bowling

There are two main ways to aim in bowling—pin bowling and spot bowling. **Pin bowling**, used primarily by novice bowlers, is little more than sighting at the pins at the end of the lane. **Spot bowling**, which has been found to be the most successful and accurate method, is aiming at the target arrows 15 feet in front of the foul line.

Of the two, spot bowling is the preferred method of aiming due to the consistency it promotes. Consistency is very important in the game of bowling, and aiming is no exception. In spot bowling for **right-handed bowlers**, the second and third target arrows from the right will be the constant targets (Figure 2.9A).

For **left-handed bowlers**, it will be the second and third arrows from the left (Figure 2.9B).

What are the advantages of **spot bowling**? First of all, it is undeniably easier to hit a target 15 feet away than one 60 feet away. Secondly, all bowling lanes are constructed the same, so the bowler has a uniform place to focus the eyes and make rational adjustments. Spot bowling also creates a better approach form by keeping a more balanced finishing position. Finally it assists with the follow-through motion of the release by giving the bowler something to reach toward with the extended delivery arm.

Pin Placement in Relation to Target Arrows

It has been previously established that the pins are set in a perfect 36-inch triangle on the pin deck. We have also

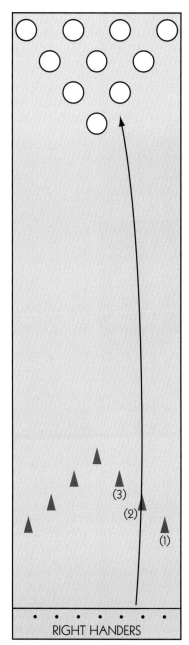

FIGURE 2.9A   Right Handers—During spot bowling, the second arrow from the right becomes the prime target.

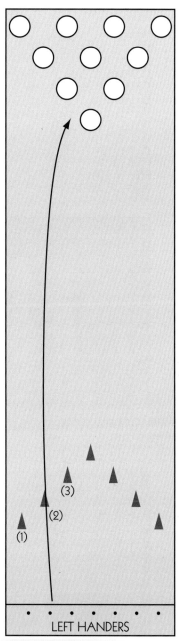

FIGURE 2.9B   Left Handers—During spot bowling, the second arrow from the left becomes the prime target.

Self Evaluation QUESTIONS

1. How many boards apart are the pins?
2. Do they line up with the target arrows and locator dots?
3. On which board do we find the following:
   a. Head pin
   b. 2 pin
   c. 3 pin
   d. 1-3 pocket
   e. 1-2 pocket for left handers

noted that the lane is made up of 39 boards with the head pin centered on the 20th board. Keep in mind that the pins are 12 inches apart from center to center. Also remember that the target arrows on the lane and all of the locator dots on the approach are spaced 5 boards apart.

Note: Because the pins are 5½ boards apart, it should be noted that the target arrows *do not* line up with the pins. Therefore, for **right-handed bowlers**, the head pin is located on the 20th board; the 2 pin is near the 26th board; and the 3 pin is sitting near the 14th board (Figure 6.1). With this in mind, one sees that the right hander's pocket for a **"perfect" strike** is halfway between the head pin and 3 pin (1–3) or the 17th board. The **"Brooklyn"** pocket for right handers (the less desirable strike pocket) is between the head pin and the 2 pin. *Remember:* The right side of the lane is for right handers and they count boards and target arrows starting from the right-hand channel toward the left.

The left side of the lane is for left handers, and they count boards and target arrows starting from the left-hand edge. The **left hander's "perfect" strike pocket** is the 1-2 pocket. Therefore, if the head pin is on the 20th board, the 2 pin would be near the 14th board from the left. Therefore, counting the boards from left to right, the 1–2 pocket is on the 17th board. Crossing over to the 1–3 pocket would be the 23rd board (Figure 2.10).

Perfect Strike Pin Action

It is every bowler's dream to roll a perfect game of 300, which is stringing twelve strikes in a row. Such an accomplishment is elusive at best. To obtain the **perfect strike**, in comparison to a "sloppy" or "lucky" strike, it

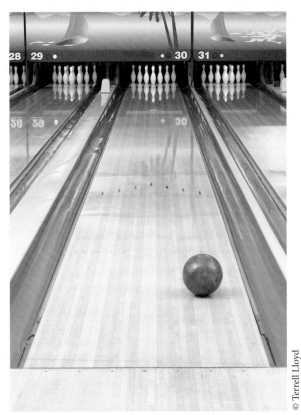

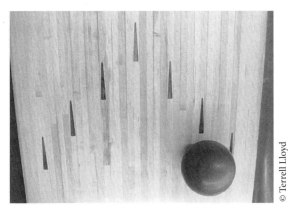

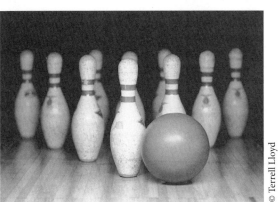

FIGURE 2.10A   Right Handers. To achieve a perfect strike, the ball must cross the 17th board at an angle. Delivering the ball across the second arrow helps to accomplish this.

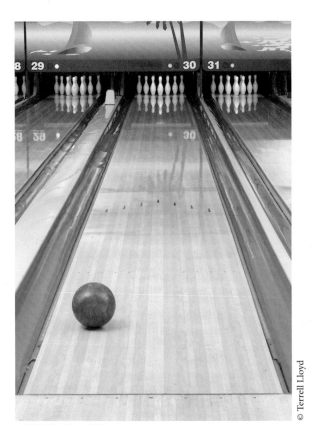

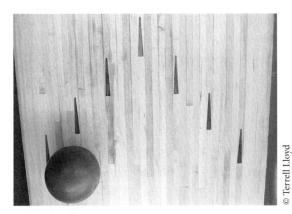

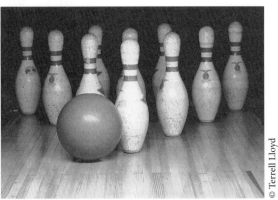

FIGURE 2.10B   Left Handers. To achieve a perfect strike, the ball must cross the 17th board at an angle. Delivering the ball across the second arrow helps to accomplish this.

is an absolute necessity for the ball to roll into that perfect strike pocket at the proper angle.

Right Handers: In a perfect strike, the ball only contacts four pins on its way through to the pit area—the 1, 3, 5, and 9 pins. The rest of the pinfall is due to a chain reaction of falling pins. If the ball's angle of entry is exact, hitting the correct impact point on the head pin, the result will be the head pin falling into the 2 pin, the 2 pin falling to the 4, and the 4 pin hitting the 7 pin. This row of pins (1, 2, 4, 7) is called the **"accuracy line"** of pins. As a result of hitting the correct impact point on the 3 pin, it will fall in the opposite direction, taking out the 6 pin, with the 6 pin hitting the 10 pin. This line of pins (3, 6, 10) is called the **"carry line."** The ball with its driving action should contact the 5 pin, which in turn falls into the 8 pin. Finally, the ball itself hits the 9 pin (Figure 2.11A).

Left Handers: In a perfect strike, the ball only contacts four pins on its way through to the pit area—the 1, 2, 5, and 8 pins. The rest of the pinfall is due to a chain reaction of falling pins. If the ball's angle of entry is exact, hitting the correct impact point on the head pin, the result will be the head pin falling into the 3 pin, the 3 pin falling into the 6 pin, and the 6 pin falling into the 10 pin. This row of pins (1, 3, 6, 10) is known as the left hander's "accuracy line." As a result of hitting the correct impact point on the 2 pin, the 2 pin will fall in the opposite direction taking out the 4 pin, and the 4 pin then takes out the 7 pin. This pin fall is called the "carry line." The ball contacts the 1, 2, 5, and 8 pins. The 5 pin takes out the 9 pin (Figure 2.11B).

This entire successive domino action results in a "perfect" strike. It is a result of the ball entering the pocket on the exact board, at the exact angle, with sufficient ball weight and enough roll to avoid undue ball deflection.

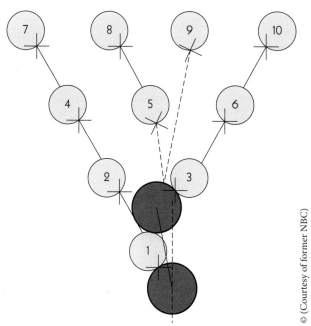

© (Courtesy of former NBC)

FIGURE 2.11A Right Handers. The ball and pin action in a perfect strike.

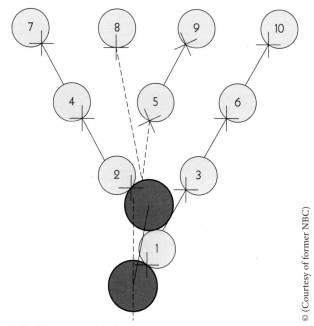

© (Courtesy of former NBC)

FIGURE 2.11B Left Handers. The ball and pin action in a perfect strike.

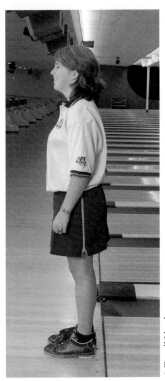

FIGURE 2.12 To find the starting distance from the foul line, place heels two to three inches away from the foul line.

© Terrell Lloyd

Starting Position

Now that we have a basic understanding of what our bowling ball is supposed to accomplish as it hits the pins, it is now time to examine possibly the most important part of one's bowling technique, the starting position on the approach.

Note: Because the four-step approach is the easiest approach to learn and in order to get some semblance of timing, rhythm, and a feeling for the movement of the ball, we will be presenting everything from a four-step basis.

In order to find a place on the approach as a **point of origin or starting position,** two questions must be answered: (1) How far from the foul line should the stance be taken to start the approach, and (2) on which dot or board should the feet be placed in order to roll the ball over the second target arrow?

To find the distance from the foul line, a bowler should go to the foul line and turn his or her back to the pins. The heels are placed in front of the locator dots (Figure 2.12). While keeping the eyes focused on the far wall, the bowler either takes three steps and a slide or four steps plus another half step toward the end of the approach area. The spot where the last foot ended will mark the correct starting distance from the line. This position may be adjusted slightly as need arises. Most bowlers of an average height and average temperament will end up around the 12-foot line.

The distance may vary from individual to individual due to: (1) the length of the legs, (2) the height of the individual, and (3) the type of personality (e.g., the active person will take livelier and longer steps than the slow, easy-going person).

The second assessment that must be made concerns the lateral placement of the feet on the approach. The exact board from which a bowler should start is, again, somewhat individualistic because it depends upon the shoulder and hip width of the individual. The best measurement for a **right-handed** bowler is to stand far enough left on the approach so the right arm, hanging at the side, is in direct line with the target arrow, which is also the locator dots corresponding to the 10th board. In this position the bowler's hips and shoulders are "square" to the aiming point. Looking down at the inside edge of the left shoe (right handers), note the exact location of the inside edge of that foot. This will be your starting position and should remain constant in order for you to gain accuracy and consistency (Figure 2.13A).

The best measurement for a **left-handed bowler** is to stand far enough right on the approach so the left arm, hanging at the side, is in direct line with the target arrow corresponding to the 10th board from the left. In this position the bowler's hips and shoulders are "square" to the aiming point. Looking down at the inside edge of the right shoe (left handers), note the exact location of the inside edge of that foot. This will be your starting position and should remain constant in order for you to gain accuracy and consistency (Figure 2.13B).

Self Evaluation QUESTIONS ?

1. What are the two impact points for a perfect strike (right and left handers)?

2. In the following diagram of the pins, show the ball and pin action for a perfect strike. (Indicate whether right- or left-handed.)

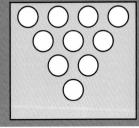

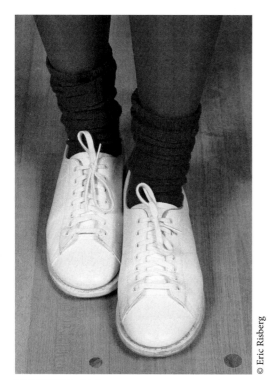

© Eric Risberg

FIGURE 2.13A   Right Handers—Check the exact location of the inside edge of the left foot in the stance position.

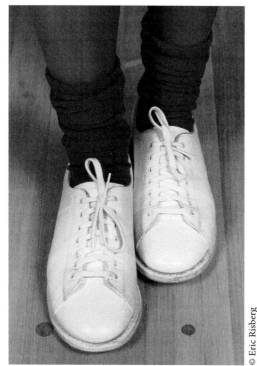

© Eric Risberg

FIGURE 2.13B   Left Handers—Check the exact location of the inside edge of the right foot in the stance position.

In Preparing for Action We Have Now Found:

- The bowling ball should be the proper weight and fit.
- There are two main methods of aiming—pin bowling and spot bowling—but the most accurate and easiest to learn of the two is spot bowling.
- The ball only strikes 4 pins in a perfect strike. The remaining pins are a result of pin action and deflection.
- Proper foot placement for the stance point of origin is twofold:
  (1) distance from the foul line and
  (2) lateral placement to line up the bowling arm with the second target arrow.

Right-handed bowlers only:

- Right-handed bowlers should wear right-handed player shoes.
- For a perfect strike to occur, the ball must enter the 1–3 pocket at an angle and be equidistant between the 1 and 3 pin.
- The pins are spaced approximately 5½ boards apart so the 1–3 pocket is halfway between the pins or three boards to the right of the head pin, or the 17th board.
- To roll a hook ball, the ball is held with the thumb at the 10 o'clock position and the fingers at 4 o'clock.
- In spot bowling, the second and third target arrows from the right, found approximately 15 feet in front of the foul line, are the point of aim for right-handed bowlers.

Left-handed bowlers only:

- Left-handed bowlers should wear left-handed player shoes.
- For a perfect strike to occur, the ball must enter the 1–2 pocket at an angle and be equidistant between the 1 and 2 pin.
- The pins are spaced approximately 5½ boards apart so the 1–2 pocket is halfway between the pins, or three boards to the left of the head pin, 17th board from the left.
- To roll a hook ball, the ball is held with the thumb at the 2 o'clock position and the fingers at 8 o'clock.
- In spot bowling, the second and third arrows from the left, found approximately 15 feet in front of the foul line, are the point of aim for left-handed bowlers.

Hints for Success

- While a partner supports the ball, place your thumb and fingers in it. Now place a pencil under the palm of your hand. If the finger span is correct, the pencil will not slide out easily (Figure 2.14).
- While the ball rests on a solid surface, insert your thumb and fingers. If it is a proper fit, a friend can tuck a little finger under the palm (Figure 2.15).
- As you release, shake hands with the target arrow (Figure 2.16A and 2.16B).
- Visualize gripping a suitcase handle with your thumb to the left (left handers, thumb is to the

Self Evaluation QUESTIONS

1. How far back on the approach should you stand?
2. How do you measure this?
3. How do you know where your left foot should be placed in your stance?
4. How many steps are recommended for the approach?

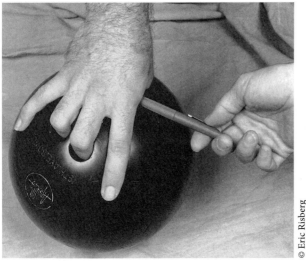

© Eric Risberg

FIGURE 2.14 Placing a pen or pencil under the palm is a way to check the span.

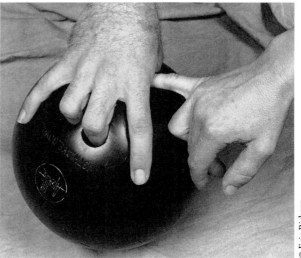

© Eric Risberg

FIGURE 2.15 Inserting the little finger under the palm is another way to check the span.

right). Now on your swing and delivery, keep the thumb and fingers in that same position and do not let the suitcase go broadside to the target at any point in the swing (Figure 2.17).

● Observe your wrist when holding the ball. It should be straight without any wrinkles on the inside or outside of it (Figure 2.18).

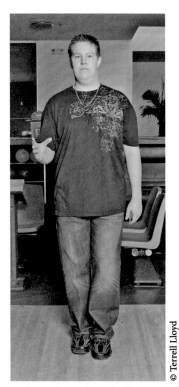

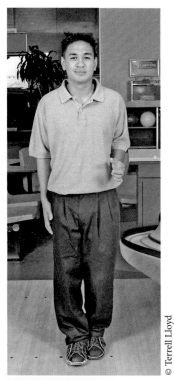

FIGURE 2.16A   Right Handers—You can attain the proper hand position by visualizing that you are shaking hands with the target.

FIGURE 2.16B   Left Handers—You can attain the proper hand position by visualizing that you are shaking hands with the target.

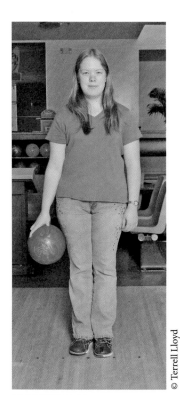

FIGURE 2.17   The thumb should be facing toward the body during the swing.

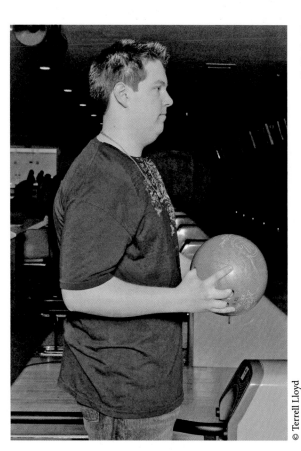

FIGURE 2.18   In the stance and swing, a straight wrist should be maintained.

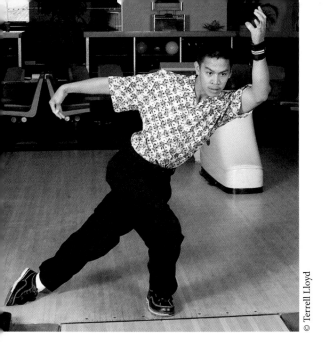
© Terrell Lloyd

3

Stance, Approach, and Delivery Concepts

Because most of the errors in bowling are directly related to the approach, it is imperative that a basic approach model be developed that uses concepts applicable to everyone. Of the millions of bowlers in the world, no two bowlers bowl exactly the same way. This is due to many variables, such as the difference in personalities, body structure, strength, and motivation. Sometimes it is very difficult to distinguish between a person's style and those principles and concepts that are common to all good bowlers.

There are at least four fundamental concepts that apply to all bowlers—good flexibility, balance, timing, and direction. All bowlers need to incorporate these concepts into their game through the practice of efficient movement principles. In this developmental process, the goal should be the fluid integration of the mechanical principles while acquiring a natural feeling for the rhythm of the approach and delivery.

Flexibility and Stance

Once the point of origin for the approach has been established, it is important that the body assume a flexible position before starting the approach. This flexibility in the beginning will follow the bowler throughout the entire delivery and, once lost, cannot be retrieved. **Flexibility** is ensured by making several conscious body adjustments in the stance position. **For right handers** to prepare for a four-step approach, the bowler should place the left foot slightly forward of the right so that the toe of the right foot is somewhere near the instep of the left foot. The feet are parallel and about two inches apart (Figure 3.1A). The mass of the body weight should be shifted to the ball of the left foot. These two actions will result in a bowler automatically stepping out with the right foot, eliminating the worry of which foot steps first.

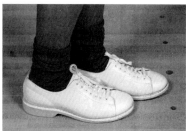
© Eric Risberg

FIGURE 3.1A Right hander— The placement of the toe of the right foot opposite the instep of the left foot.

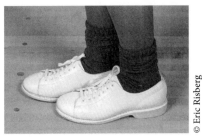

© Eric Risberg

FIGURE 3.1B   Left hander— The placement of the toe of the left foot opposite the instep of the right foot.

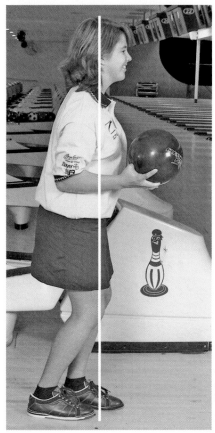

© Terrell Lloyd

FIGURE 3.2   The vertical balance line in the stance.

For left handers to prepare for a four-step approach, the bowler should place the right foot slightly forward of the left so the toe of the left foot is somewhere near the instep of the right foot. The feet are parallel and about two inches apart (Figure 3.1B). The mass of the body weight should be shifted to the ball of the right foot. These two actions will result in a bowler automatically stepping out with the left foot, eliminating the worry of which foot steps forward first.

The most important ingredient in our flexibility concept is the establishment of a small degree of flexion in the knees. It is this knee flexion that allows all other things to happen correctly. To maintain good body balance, the bowler should lean forward slightly from the hips, keeping the back relatively straight.

Balance and the Stance

Good balance is a very important aspect of bowling. The **vertical balance line** can be found in an upright body simply by drawing an imaginary straight line from the shoulders through the knees perpendicular to the floor. The more the knees bend, the more the shoulders have to tilt forward for the body to remain in balance. When a bowler is balanced, he or she will feel comfortable (Figure 3.2).

The ball should be supported in the non-bowling hand until the point of origin on the approach is reached. When ready to assume the stance position, insert the fingers into the ball, followed by the thumb. The thumb should be inserted all the way to the webbing. Then, roll the ball from the non-bowling hand to the bowling hand. **Right handers** will have the thumb and fingers at the 10 and 4 o'clock position. It is recommended that the right-handed bowler hold the ball toward the right side of the body, approximately at waist level with the right forearm resting on the hip (Figure 3.3).

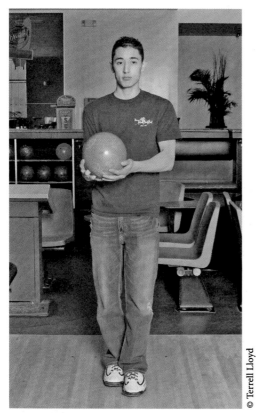

FIGURE 3.3   Right Hander—Holding the ball off to the right side of the body.

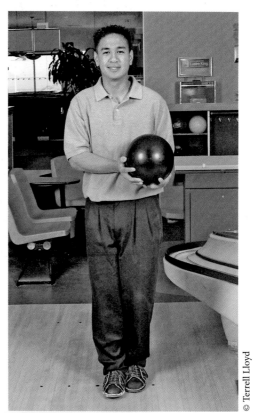

FIGURE 3.4   Left Hander—Holding the ball off to the left side of the body.

Left handers should insert their thumb and fingers at 2 and 8 o'clock position and hold the ball to the left side of the body, approximately at waist level with the left forearm resting on the hip (Figure 3.4).

Many problems will stem from a ball held in the center of the body, primarily because the ball must be swung out and around to clear the hips. This would result in an inconsistent round-house swing, a swing that goes out and away from the body. Because it is important to keep everything in a straight line, holding the ball to the right locates it properly for the pendular swing pattern.

If the ball does not feel comfortable at waist height, it may be adjusted anywhere between the waist and shoulder as long as it remains slightly to the side of the body (Figures 3.3 and 3.4). If held at shoulder height, the elbows would be resting on the hips (Figure 3.5). In this position, the ball is found near the balance line regardless of whether it is waist or shoulder high. When balanced, the ball will not feel as heavy as it would if held in front of the bowler outside the balance line. Again, it should feel comfortable. We are well on the way to a good approach when we have established a balanced stance position with a degree of flexibility (Figure 3.6).

Self Evaluation
QUESTIONS

1. What are the ingredients of a good stance?

2. How can flexibility be introduced into the stance?

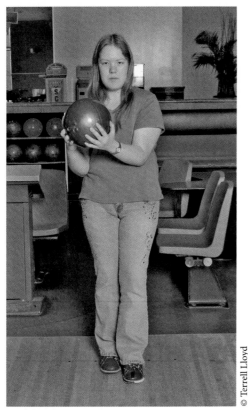

FIGURE 3.5   The ball at shoulder level in the stance.

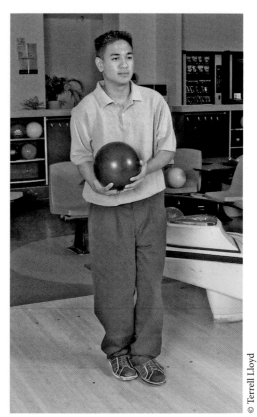

FIGURE 3.6   In the stance, the bowler should maintain a balanced and flexible position.

Timing and Pushaway

The most important part of the bowling approach is the pushaway. It creates timing for the entire approach, swing, and delivery. The **pushaway** is the movement of the ball away from the body, which sets the approach and the swing in motion.

The key feature of this concept is that the ball initiates all movement. The ball is moved approximately 3 inches outward and downward to a point where the elbow straightens. The left hand leaves the ball at the end of the pushaway movement. At this point, the balance line of the stance has been intentionally destroyed. Because an unbalanced position has been assumed, the bowler

will tilt further forward and react by taking a step, to keep the body from falling forward (Figures 3.7 and 3.8). This cause-and-effect motion will always happen at the same (redundant) point, consistently and automatically.

The length of the first step is in direct relationship to the length of the pushaway. The farther out the ball is pushed, the longer the first step will be. It is recommended that the first step be fairly short, to maintain a forward flex of the body. If the pushaway goes up and out, it will force a longer first step, causing the body to lean backward, resulting in the loss of good vertical line and flexibility.

To check for proper timing of the swing in relation to the steps,

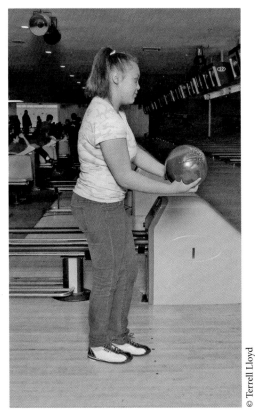

FIGURE 3.7 The pushaway initiates all movement in the approach.

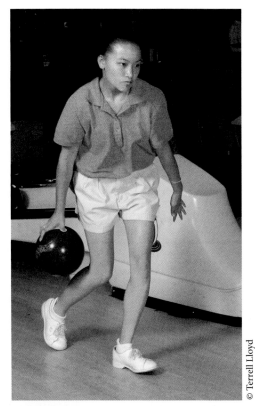

FIGURE 3.8 The downward direction of the pushaway showing the straightening of the elbow.

© Terrell Lloyd

© Terrell Lloyd

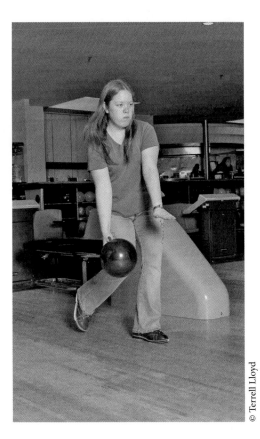

FIGURE 3.9 The point to best check for proper swing and foot coordination is on the second step. The ball should be in the downward position.

© Terrell Lloyd

the second step should be observed. On the second step, the ball should be straight down in the swing (Figure 3.9).

Remember: Move the ball out and in a downward direction and let the feet follow the natural urge to put the body into motion.

Flexibility and Balance in the Approach

The flexibility and balance obtained in the stance should follow-throughout the entire approach. To maintain the **vertical balance line** in the approach, flex the knees and take shuffling steps on the balls of the feet instead of using walking steps with a heel–toe action. A **shuffle** is merely a graceful gliding or skating motion across the surface of the approach. This gliding action prevents the body from bouncing up and down and breaking the rhythm of the approach and swing.

The four-step approach is really three shuffles and a slide. With each shuffle the knees progressively increase their flexion, allowing the body and the ball to be progressively lowered toward the floor for a smooth delivery (Figure 3.10).

Direction in the Approach and Delivery

The last concept in the approach model is **direction**. This concept includes achieving direction toward the target, accuracy in terms of the release, a complete follow-through, and the finishing position.

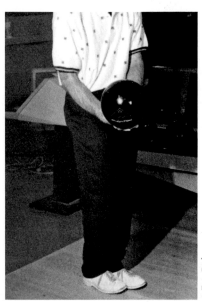
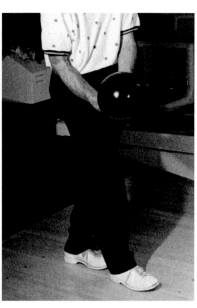
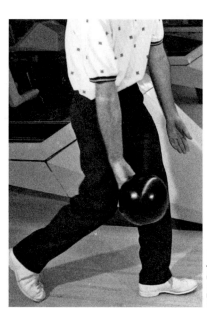

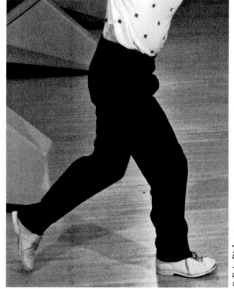
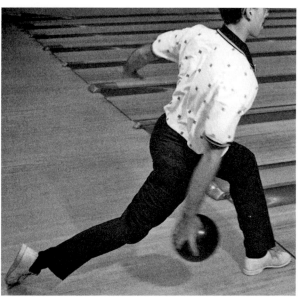

FIGURE 3.10
Showing the increased knee flexion during the entire approach.

A good swing will have the following ingredients resulting in the needed accuracy:

- The ball should swing through a natural pendular arc at its own rate of speed. The speed of the swing is directly related to the length of the arm and the weight of the ball.
- The height of the arc in the backswing should equal the height of the pushaway.
- The arm should follow the natural swing of the ball. The bowler adjusts the rate of the steps to the swing rather than intentionally tampering with the pendular swing in order to match the feet.
- The pendular swing should remain in a straight line with the elbow "grazing" the hip as it moves back and forth.
- On the downswing going into the release, a slight acceleration often occurs, providing extra impetus to the "lift" and rotation mechanism at the point of release.

The Release

Right handers: For the beginning bowler the release is very simple. The 10–4 o'clock position (2–8 o'clock for left handers) that was established in the stance is maintained throughout the swing and is still present in the finishing position (Figure 3.11).

The wrist remains firm and straight and the forearm rotates minimally in the swing and release. The

FIGURE 3.11

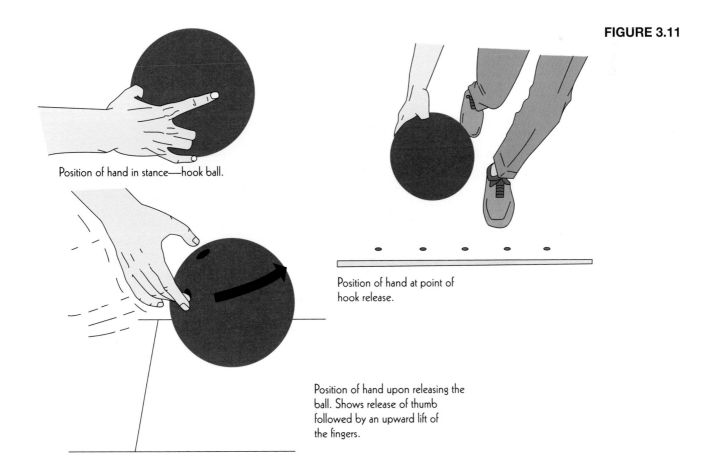

Position of hand in stance—hook ball.

Position of hand at point of hook release.

Position of hand upon releasing the ball. Shows release of thumb followed by an upward lift of the fingers.

sliding foot should point toward the target (Figure 3.12A).

As the ball is released on the far side of the foul line, the thumb should come out of the ball before the fingers, allowing the lifting action of the fingers in the 4 o'clock position to occur as the ball starts upward in the pendular swing (Figures 3.13 and 3.14). This creates a force off the center of the ball that results in a right-to-left rotation of the ball. The resultant ball roll will find the ball going straight approximately

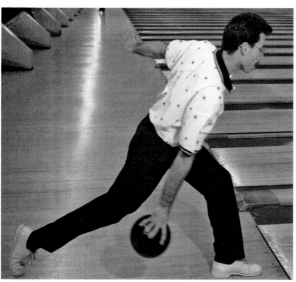

FIGURE 3.12A The 10–4 o'clock position should be held throughout the swing and delivery; the wrist remains firm and straight, and the sliding foot points toward the target.

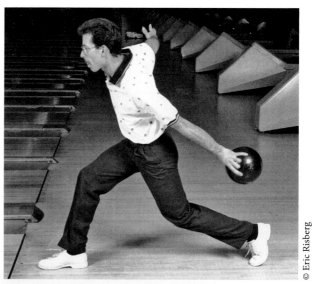

FIGURE 3.12B For a left-handed bowler, the 2–8 o'clock position should be held throughout the swing and delivery.

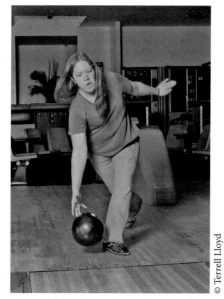

FIGURE 3.13 The thumb exits the ball before the fingers release the ball.

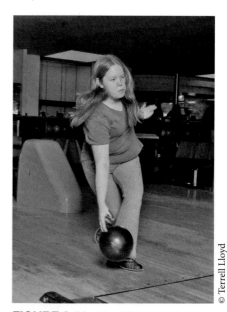

FIGURE 3.14 The "lift" placed on the ball as it is released while the arm continues upward into the follow-through.

two-thirds of the way down the lane and then, due to the frictional forces equalizing, the ball will start hooking from right to left (left handers, from left to right). This action allows the ball to be rolled over the second arrow (10th board) and hook into the 1–3 pocket (1–2 pocket for left handers) (17th board) at the proper angle (Figure 3.15).

Please Note: A hook ball is *not* achieved by rotating your hand and/or arm upon delivery. It is straight up lift and your elbow stays close to your body—*not* flailing outward.

Left handers: For the beginning left-handed bowler, the release is very simple. The 2–8 o'clock position that was established in the stance is maintained throughout the swing and is still present in the finishing position. The wrist remains firm and straight and the forearm rotates minimally in the swing and release. The sliding foot should point toward the target (Figure 3.12B). As the ball is released on the far side of the foul line, the thumb should come out of the ball before the fingers, allowing the lifting action of the fingers in the 8 o'clock position to occur as the ball starts upward in the pendular swing (Figures 3.13 and 3.14). This creates a force off the center of the ball that results in a left-to-right rotation of the ball. The resultant ball roll will find the ball going straight approximately two-thirds of the way down the lane and then, due to the frictional forces equalizing, the ball will start hooking from left to right. This action allows the ball to be rolled over the second arrow (10th board from the left) and hooking into the 1–2 pocket (17th board) at the proper angle.

The Follow-through

The last factor that assists in achieving good direction is the **extension or follow-through**. A good extension (follow-through) will find the bowler's eyes still focusing on the target and the straightened bowling arm moving forward in direct line with the target arrow (Figure 3.15).

Self Evaluation QUESTIONS?

1. What initiates the forward motion of the body?
2. Where is the ball moved in the pushaway phase?
3. With each shuffle, what happens to the knees?
4. In what position are the thumb and fingers held throughout the swing and delivery?
5. What happens at the delivery with the thumb? The fingers?
6. On which target arrow should the ball roll?

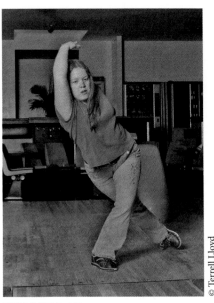

© Terrell Lloyd

FIGURE 3.15 The follow-through.

Vertical Balance Line and the Delivery

Throughout the stance and the approach, the shoulders are kept over flexed knees for the maintenance of good balance. This already established **vertical balance line** is also very important in a bowler's finishing position to allow a smooth and consistent delivery. By bending the knees rather than bending at the waist or dropping the shoulders, the bowler can get closer to the floor, which aids in placing the ball on the lane rather than dropping it (Figure 3.16). After a well-balanced delivery, the body can maintain a comfortable follow-through position (Figure 3.17).

Horizontal Balance Line and the Finish Position

Besides the vertical balance line, there is also a proper **horizontal balance line** that is critical in the finish position. To counterbalance the weight of the bowling ball that is moving in front and to the side of the body, the body must make other adjustments. The opposite arm becomes a counterbalance by being stretched out and angled a little backwards. This procedure assists in keeping the shoulders and hips square to the target.

Right handers: The most crucial adjustment for horizontal balance at the delivery is accomplished for right-handed bowlers by stretching the right leg backwards in a straightened position and letting it drift to the left in a pigeon-toed position. Turning the toe inward in this pigeon-toed position causes the hip to curl under, opening the right side (Figure 3.18A). This allows the ball to swing in an unobstructed straight line toward the target. Caution should be taken here because if the leg is kicked around behind, it will jerk the torso out of alignment. To prevent this from happening, the bowler should try to keep the toe on the approach and let it slide into place.

Left handers: The most crucial adjustment for horizontal balance at the delivery for a left hander is accomplished by stretching the left leg backwards in a straightened position and letting it drift to the right in a pigeon-toed position. Turning the toe inward in this pigeon-toed position causes the hip to curl under,

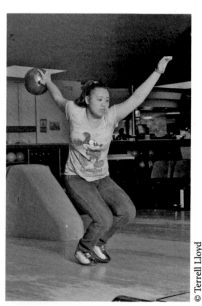

FIGURE 3.16   Increased knee flexion lowers the body to the necessary delivery level.

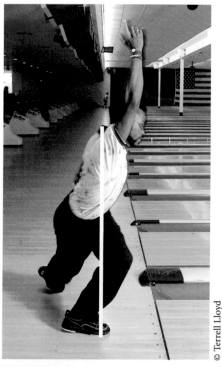

© Terrell Lloyd

FIGURE 3.17   The vertical balance line is maintained throughout the delivery and follow-through.

© Terrell Lloyd

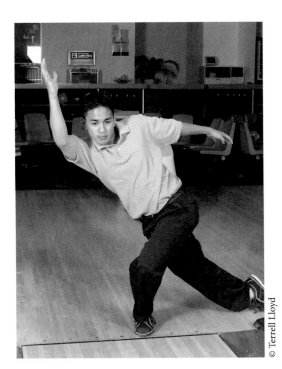
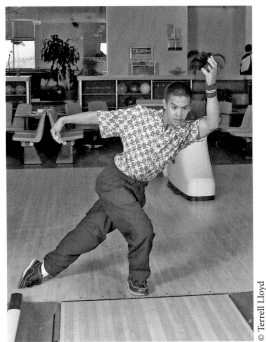

FIGURE 3.18A, B
Counterbalancing the weight of the ball by extending the opposite arm (horizontal balance).

© Terrell Lloyd

opening the left side (Figure 3.18B). This allows the ball to swing in an unobstructed straight line toward the target. Caution should be taken here because if the leg is kicked around behind, it will jerk the torso out of alignment. To prevent this from happening, the bowler should try to keep the toe on the approach and let it slide into place.

Hand and Arm Position in the Follow-through

After the ball has been delivered, the bowling arm continues to move forward in a direct line with the target arrow. The finish position should find a 90-degree angle formed between the shoulder, the arm, and the target

with the fingers curled into the palm of the hand. The eyes remain focused on the target arrow and should be able to identify the exact board over which the ball is rolled.

Self Evaluation QUESTIONS?

1. How is the body lowered in order to lay the ball on the floor in the delivery?

2. What body adjustment must be made to counterbalance the weight of the ball in the approach? The delivery?

3. Explain the action of the trailing leg in the delivery.

4. Explain the finish position of the arms and fingers.

Summary of Bowling Fundamentals for Right-handed Bowlers (Figures 3.19 and 3.20)

Stance

- The left foot is placed slightly forward of the right with the majority of the body weight on the ball of the left foot.

- The knees are unlocked and slightly flexed. The shoulders are tilted forward slightly from the hips and should be directly above the knees.
- The ball is supported in the non-bowling hand until the point of origin is found and the stance has been assumed.
- The thumb and fingers of the bowling hand are now inserted into the ball (fingers first) at the 10 and 4 o'clock position. Then it is rolled from the non-bowling hand to the bowling hand.

FIGURE 3.19
A side angle view of a four-step approach.

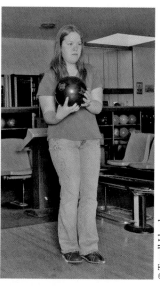
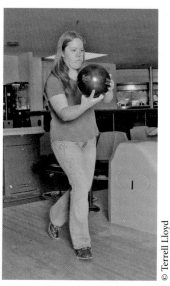
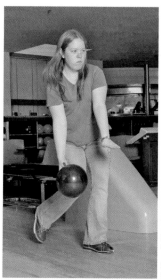
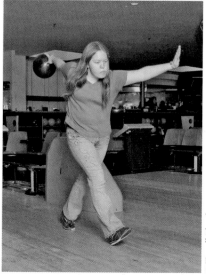
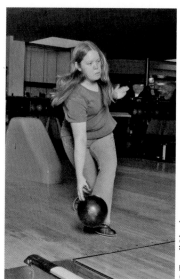
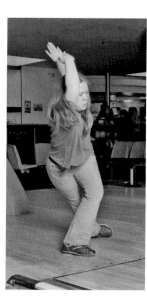

© Terrell Lloyd

- The ball is held to the right front of the body at approximately waist height with the forearm resting on the hip. The ball is near the vertical balance line drawing a line through the shoulders and knees and is supported slightly by the non-bowling hand.
- The shoulders and hips should be square to the intended line of ball roll.

Pushaway

- The most crucial part of the approach and swing is in timing the pushaway with the approach.
- The pushaway is a movement of the ball out from the body in a downward direction resulting in the straightening of the bowling arm.
- The pushaway action puts the body in an unbalanced position and will cause the body to take a step forward.
- The step forward will be with the right foot, which was the unweighted back foot in the stance.

Approach

- During the approach, the feet will take three shuffle steps and a slide.
- Each shuffle step will find the knees progressively more flexed.
- The shuffle should be in a straight line moving toward the target arrow.
- The eyes of the bowler are focused solely on the target.
- If the swing and the approach are coordinated, the ball will be just starting to move upward into the backswing on the second step.

Swing

- The weight of the ball straightens the elbow on the pushaway that is the start of the arc for the pendular swing.
- The ball swings straight back in the natural pendular swing to the height of the backswing, somewhere between the waist and the shoulder.
- During this swing the 10–4 o'clock thumb-finger position is maintained with a straight elbow and firm wrist.
- The wrist remains firm through the swing, including the peak backswing position.
- The shoulders and hips are square to the target throughout the swing.
- The non-bowling arm is extended to the side and slightly back for balance.

Delivery

- The slide is accomplished by bending the knees to the point where the ball can swing out on the lane without being dropped or dropping the shoulder.
- The shoulders are moved forward from the hips and aligned directly over the knees, to keep the vertical balance line intact.
- To counterbalance the weight of the ball that has moved in front of the vertical balance line, the right leg is extended back and drifts to the left in a pigeon-toed fashion.
- The hips and shoulders remain square to the target.
- The ball is released on the far side of the foul line as it starts upward in the pendular swing.
- On the release, the thumb and fingers are still in the 10–4 o'clock position.
- The thumb is automatically released from the ball first and then the fingers are released with an upward lifting action. The off-center lift will cause the ball to have a right-to-left (counterclockwise) rotation, resulting in a slight hook.

Follow-through

- The eyes remain focused on the target arrow.
- The bowling arm moves forward in a direct line with the target arrow.
- The fingers are curled toward the palm of the hand.
- The finish position is a 90-degree angle formed between the shoulder, the arm, and the target.

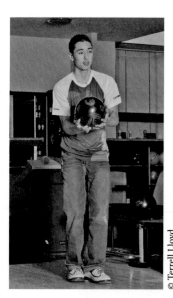
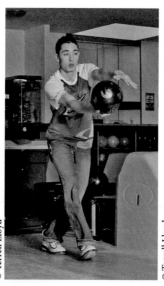
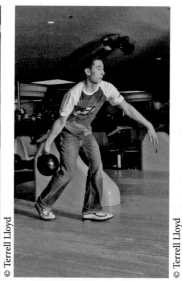
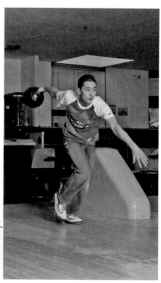

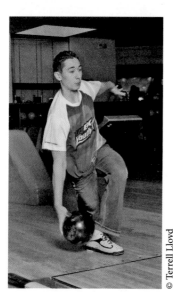
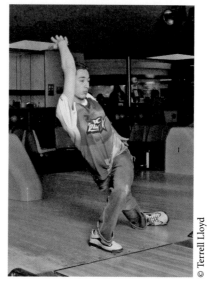

FIGURE 3.20   A side angle view of a four-step approach.

Summary of Bowling Fundamentals for Left-handed Bowlers (Figure 3.21)

Stance

- The right foot is placed forward of the left with the majority of the body weight on the ball of the right foot.
- The knees are unlocked and slightly flexed. The shoulders are tilted forward slightly from the hips and should be directly over the knees.
- The ball is supported in the right hand while taking position at the point of origin.
- The thumb and fingers of the bowling hand are now inserted into the ball at the 2 and 8 o'clock position, fingers first. Then the ball is rolled from the non-bowling hand to the bowling hand.
- The ball is held to the left front of the body at approximately waist height with the forearm resting on the hip. The ball is near the vertical balance line drawing a line through the shoulders and knees and is supported slightly by the non-bowling hand.
- The shoulders and hips should be square to the intended line of the ball roll.

Pushaway

- The crucial part of the approach and swing is in timing the pushaway with the approach.
- The pushaway is a movement of the ball out from the body in a downward direction resulting in the straightening of the bowling arm.
- The pushaway action puts the body in an unbalanced position and will cause the body to take a step forward.
- The step forward will be with the left foot, which was the unweighted back foot in the stance.

Approach

- During the approach, the feet will take three shuffle steps and a slide.
- Each shuffle step finds the knees progressively more flexed.
- The shuffle should be in a straight line moving toward the target arrow.
- The eyes of the bowler are focused solely on the target.
- If the swing and the approach are coordinated, the ball will be just starting to move upward into the backswing on the second step.

Swing

- The weight of the ball straightens the elbow on the pushaway, which is the start of the arc for the pendular swing.
- The ball swings straight back in the natural pendular swing to the height of the backswing, somewhere between the waist and shoulders.
- During this swing, the 2–8 o'clock thumb-finger position is maintained with a straight elbow and firm wrist.
- The wrist remains firm throughout the swing, including the peak backswing position.
- The non-bowling arm (right) is extended to the side and slightly back for balance.

Delivery

- The slide is accomplished by bending the knee to the point where the ball can swing out on the lane without being dropped or dropping the shoulder.

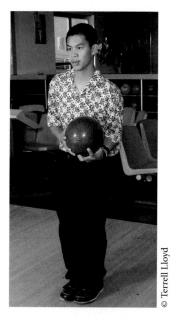
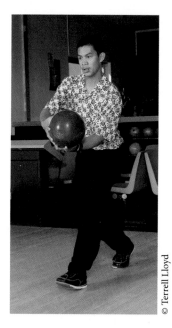
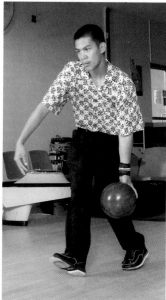

© Terrell Lloyd

© Terrell Lloyd

© Terrell Lloyd

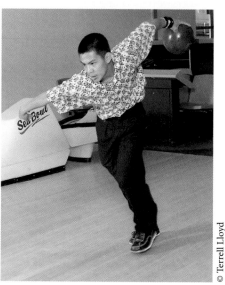
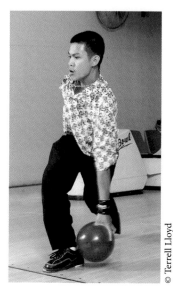
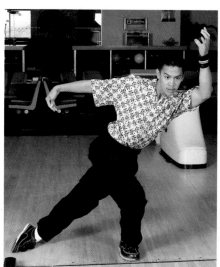

© Terrell Lloyd

© Terrell Lloyd

© Terrell Lloyd

FIGURE 3.21   A front view of a four-step approach.

- The shoulders are moved forward from the hips and aligned directly over the knees to keep the vertical line intact.
- To counterbalance the weight of the ball that has moved in front of the vertical balance line, the left leg is extended back and drifts to the right in a pigeon-toed fashion.
- The hips and shoulders remain square to the target.
- The ball is released on the far side of the foul line as it starts upward in the pendular swing.

- On the release, the thumb and fingers are still in the 2–8 o'clock position.
- The thumb is automatically released from the ball first and then the fingers are released with an upward lifting action. The off-center lift will cause the ball to have a left-to-right (clockwise) rotation, resulting in a slight hook.

Follow-through

- The eyes remain focused on the target arrow until the ball passes over the target.
- The bowling arm moves forward in a direct line with the target arrow.

- The fingers are curled toward the palm of the hand.
- The finish position is a 90-degree angle formed between the shoulder, the arm, and the target.

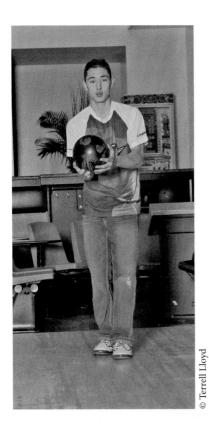

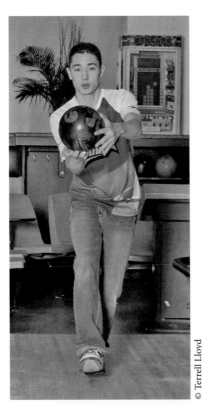

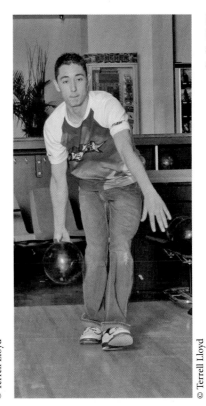

FIGURE 3.22
Front view of a four-step approach A-F.

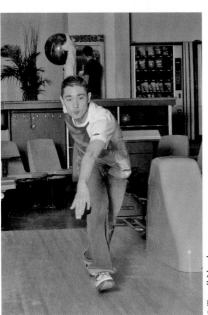

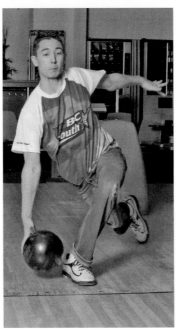

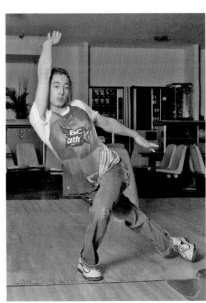

© Terrell Lloyd

Hints for Success

Approach

- To practice shuffling without the ball, try keeping your footwork quiet and noiseless. The noise should resemble sandpaper rubbing across wood.
- To increase the shuffling action, visualize "sneaking up" to the foul line.
- To maintain balance and to keep your body from bouncing during the approach, visualize approaching the line with a glass of water on each shoulder.
- To keep yourself from "drifting," visualize taking the approach on a balance beam.

Arm Swing

- To emphasize the natural pendular motion of the arm swing, visualize the arm as a pendulum on a large clock. Then take practice swings, allowing the ball to swing in a natural pendular motion and rate of speed.
- To assist in keeping the swing straight, try to feel your elbow grazing past the hip.

Ball Release

- To assist in getting more "lift," visualize squeezing a gun trigger as the ball comes off the hand in the release.

- To assist in getting more lift, feel the finger pressure in the ball and, upon release, curl the fingers into the palm of your hand.

Body Balance in the Release and Follow-through

- To assist in staying low and in balance throughout the release and follow-through, visualize extending the kneecap (not the head) over the foul line while keeping the slide foot flat on the approach.
- To ensure the proper use of the balance arm and avoid a "dropped shoulder," visualize holding a bucket of water with the left hand (left handers—right hand).

Follow-through

- To ensure a complete follow-through and correct direction, visualize holding a glass of water in the bowling hand and tossing the water up and over your shoulder, keeping the elbow straight as long as possible.
- To maintain the follow-through and body stability at the foul line, "stay still" until the ball passes the target arrow.

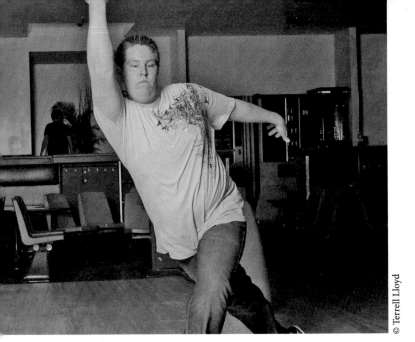

© Terrell Lloyd

4

Principles of Movement Applied to Bowling

As was previously noted, it is important to know the "whys and wherefores" when learning or trying to improve a skill. If you know the concepts and principles involved in effective movement, learning can be enhanced by making it more meaningful. Analysis and error correction then becomes second nature.

We are most likely all familiar with Newton's Law of Motion that states, "An object that is at rest or is in motion will remain at rest or in motion at the same speed, in a straight line, unless acted upon by an outside force." This principle will be our chief guide throughout our bowling swing, approach, and delivery. In analyzing each phase of this physical law, many other concepts and principles enter the picture.

Weight of the Ball

It has been previously noted that weight is an important consideration when selecting a ball. Each bowler should select a ball that is as heavy as he or she can control. The reason for this is quite obvious when one considers the principles of force and gravity. In an underarm swing pattern, gravity will cause the ball to swing in a straight, pendular fashion unless

restricted or acted upon by another force. If the ball is heavy enough, and if a bowler will allow this natural swing, force will be produced by gravity and momentum, not by the bowler "muscling" and forcing the ball. In this natural swing pattern, the direction of the swing will always remain constant and, if lined up correctly, will remain in a straight line. If the ball is too light, a bowler has the tendency to push or pull the ball off his or her natural swing line, resulting in inconsistency. Additionally, a heavier ball will usually result in greater pin fall. This is because a heavier ball does not deflect as easily as a lighter ball when it contacts the weight of the pins.

Force Production

It is essential that enough force be generated at delivery to allow the ball to travel effectively on course. Force is generated during the swing and the approach.

Swing

The production of gravitational force in the swing is directly related to the following principle: *The greater distance the swinging object travels, the more time for gravity to act on the ball,*

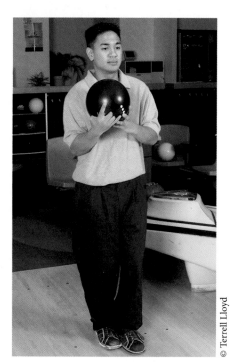

FIGURE 4.1 The ball can be held high in the stance for the production of more momentum.

thereby producing more force. Consequently, a ball held higher in the stance, all things being equal, would result in a longer arc because the backswing would equal the height of the pushaway (Figure 4.1). The ball would be traveling a greater distance, allowing gravity to have more time to act on the ball, resulting in more ball velocity at the time of delivery.

A bowler having trouble producing enough force at the delivery may want to try holding the ball higher in the stance. Gradual changes are recommended to maintain good form and consistency.

Another way of allowing the ball to travel a greater distance in the swing is to lengthen the lever that is moving through space. That lever, the bowler's arm, should be completely straightened in the pushaway and the backswing to allow for maximum length.

Because of the added weight of the ball and the momentum that the ball is gathering, the body must remain stable and firm throughout the entire swing. By stabilizing the shoulder and wrist of the swinging arm, the pendular swing will stay in a straight line. This stabilizing action will also keep the shoulder from dropping and free it from muscle strain. Stabilizing the wrist during all phases of the swing, particularly the backswing, merely keeps the ball from straying off the desired pendular path.

Approach

The main purpose of an approach is to gather the forward body momentum that will be transferred to the ball at the release. A gravitational swing alone will not build up enough momentum to roll the ball at a speed great enough to hold the desired line and successfully knock down the pins, so it is necessary to add an approach to assist in this force production.

The principle of time and distance becomes important when developing momentum in the approach. The greater the time and distance over which momentum is developed, the greater the force imparted. Therefore, the longer and faster the approach, all things being equal, the greater the momentum build-up. Many times this results in bowlers running to the foul line from the end of the approach so the ball will have greater momentum. Erroneously, they assume that this fast ball will scare the pins down. Remember, in bowling everything is controlled and coordinated. An approach should only be as long and as fast as needed to coordinate with the swing, to hold the desired line to the pins, and to knock the pins down.

Here are some factors to keep in mind while developing momentum in the approach:

- Shuffle steps will allow for a smoother approach. By keeping the body free from bouncing, all energies will be directed to building forward momentum. Outside forces acting on the ball swing will be kept to a minimum and the ball will remain in its natural arc.
- The vertical balance line should be shifted forward throughout the approach. The forward shift of body weight should be from the ankles. This helps in many ways:
  1. It will place the center of gravity in front of the pushing foot for ease in building momentum during the steps.
  2. It will assure a smooth approach by allowing the knees to act as shock absorbers in each step.
  3. It will increase the arc of the ball due to the body leaning slightly forward, allowing for greater force production.
  4. It assures the body a position over a bent knee upon release for a smooth, straight delivery.

© Terrell Lloyd

5. It forces the point of maximum momentum to coincide with the ball delivery over the foul line.

6. It allows the arm swing to continue forward for a greater distance in the follow-through for maximum momentum and direction.

It is almost impossible for a bowler who is standing erect or approaching in an erect fashion to shift his or her weight forward upon the delivery of the ball. In this erect position, the body's center of gravity is high and the body's weight is slightly back. As a result, the ball will be released beside or behind the left foot, with the swing going in an upward direction and the ball crossing the lane (Figure 4.2).

If the forward weight shift comes from the waist rather than the ankles, the hips will remain high, resulting in an unbalanced body during approach and delivery, with the majority of the force production going downward into the floor rather than out onto the lane. The resultant follow-through will be incomplete with very little chance for "lift" to be placed on the ball (Figure 4.3).

● At all times during the approach, the toes, feet, and body should be going in a straight line for maximum mechanical efficiency. This allows the feet to push directly from behind and also allows for all momentum to be directed and released in the direction of the target.

How much momentum or **ball speed** is really needed to get an effective ball roll? It should be noted that all good bowlers develop a specific optimal ball speed. Research has determined the optimal average ball speed to be delivered at 17 miles per hour, or 2.4 seconds from the point of release to the head pin. At this speed, all governing forces will be in proper balance, allowing the ball to hit the pins with the most effective impact. This speed allows the pins to topple

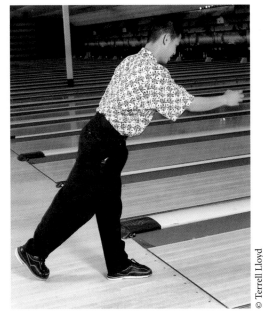

FIGURE 4.2 Releasing the ball with little knee bend usually results in a loss of accuracy.

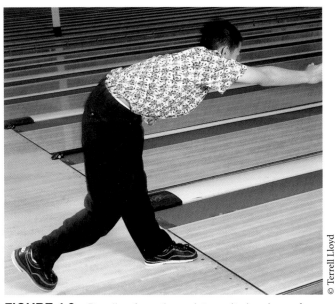

FIGURE 4.3 Bending from the waist results in a loss of power at the release point.

in a domino fashion rather than flying upward as with a fast ball. A slower ball will deflect as it hits the pins, causing ineffective pin action.

Hook Ball and Momentum

When first released, the ball is traveling at its maximum speed, and slides more than rolls in a straight line. This is partly due to the speed of the ball on the lane. Frictional forces build up between the ball and the lane and slow the ball. As the ball slows, the side rotation imparted by the fingers lifting the ball off the center of gravity (4 o'clock position for right handers and 8 o'clock for left handers) now takes effect. When this side rotation becomes greater than the forward roll, the ball begins to hook toward the pocket.

When the ball speed, forward roll, and side rotation forces are in proper balance, the result will be an effective, consistent, working hook ball.

Straight Ball Principles

Throughout this text, the authors have elected to teach only the rolling of an effective hook ball. It is the ball roll of choice, primarily due to the carrying action at the pins. However, it is foreseen that many beginning bowlers might release the ball as a straight ball with the thumb and fingers at 12 and 6 o'clock, resulting in a ball that goes straight down the lane without any side rotation. This ball roll does possess a lot of consistency and accuracy regardless of lane conditions, but it is less effective when it contacts the pins. This is primarily due to the ball deflecting away from the center pins as it contacts the first in the set. The result: the pins

behind the head pin often remain untouched.

Correction Suggestions for Straight Ball

Remember that the thumb and fingers are the problem areas that need correcting at the moment of release. The thumb and fingers are at the 12 and 6 o'clock position instead of the 10 and 4 o'clock position for right handers and the 8 and 2 o'clock position for left handers. The result: a straight ball. Two different things may be causing this finger positioning on the ball. First, the bowler might have placed his or her fingers in that position at the stance and carried it throughout the swing, approach, and delivery. Or, the bowler started with the fingers in the hook ball position and during the backswing rotated the palm of the hand down and flexed the wrist backward (as in an underhanded softball throw). The forward swing and release would probably find the fingers remaining in this 12 and 6 o'clock position and pulling up through the middle of the ball from underneath. Again, the result would be a straight ball. It is imperative that the fingers stay in the hook ball position throughout the stance, swing, and release to ensure the rotation on the ball that will result in a hook. (See the Instructor's Manual for drills and the Advanced Section of *Right Down Your Alley*.)

Backup Ball Principles

The backup ball is often referred to as a reverse hook, but it is really an offshoot of the full roller or straight ball. It hooks from right to left for right handers (left to right for left handers). It is usually due to the thumb rotating from the 10 o'clock to the 12 o'clock position (right handers) or from the 2 o'clock to the 12 o'clock position (left handers). This is an exaggeration of the straight ball release. Many bowlers continue the finger and hand rotation past the 12 o'clock position in the release. The result is a ball that rotates in a clockwise position for right handers and a counterclockwise rotation for left handers. The ball then has a reverse hooking action. This ball is fairly effective as it contacts the pins due to the ball rotation and "digging" action. However, the big drawback is the lack of consistency in the amount of the reverse hook due to the free rotation of the hand at the release point. It is difficult to release at exactly the same point of the hand rotation.

Correction Suggestions for the Backup Ball

The main correction for a backup ball is to somehow ensure that the bowler takes a hook ball finger and hand position at the time of the stance and maintains that hand position without any wrist or forearm rotation throughout the swing, approach, and delivery. At times, there is an overemphasis of the thumb and finger position by placing them at 9 and 3 o'clock (right handers) or 3 and 9 o'clock (left handers). At the release point, the bowler should try to follow-through with the index finger pointing toward the target with the fingernail facing up. This automatically puts the thumb in a 9 o'clock position (right handers) and 3 o'clock (left handers). (Additional suggestions may be found in the Instructor's Manual and in the Advanced Section of *Right Down Your Alley*.)

Correction Suggestions for Changing Ball Speeds

Any time changes are to be made in the speed of the ball, it is of great importance to maintain good coordination, flexibility, balance, and timing of the swing and approach. When a bowler is having trouble generating enough speed on the ball, it will hook too far to the left. This is due to too little slide and too much side rotation. Any of five different corrections may resolve the problem.

Not Enough Ball Speed

- The ball could be put into the swing a tad earlier to create a more rapid approach tempo.
- The ball may be held higher in the stance, which will automatically create a longer arc.
- The ball may be pushed away a bit farther on the pushaway.
- A 5-step approach may be used to give a longer approach to produce more forward momentum.

If a 5-step approach is used, the ball is held higher and pushed out a little farther for the swing to be properly coordinated.

- The approach may be started at least 6 inches further back.
- Think of reducing the overall effort put into the approach by 25 percent.
- A lighter ball could be used.

Some rethinking may be in order for those who are intent on throwing the ball as hard as they can. They are probably leaving pocket splits, often the 5 pin, and not getting effective pin action. These bowlers will continue to have these problems unless their mental attitude is changed by someone who can prove why that type of ball is not the most effective. A fast ball results in too much slide and not enough side rotation, so the hook is very minimal. The following suggestions could be considered.

Too Much Ball Speed

- In the stance, hold the ball lower to decrease the resistance of the swing.
- The pushaway could be shortened or de-emphasized.
- The knees can be flexed more because it is very difficult for anyone to move fast with flexed knees.
- Use the force of gravity to move the ball in the swing rather than forcing the ball. Flex the knees more, pushing the ball out lower, and not quite so far. This should allow the bowler to feel the natural weight of the ball swinging the arm rather than the arm doing the swinging. The bowler should constantly feel relaxed.
- The approach could be started at least 6 inches closer.

- Think of reducing the overall effort put into the approach by 25 percent.
- A heavier ball could be used.

Accuracy and Consistency Principles

Once force production is present, a bowler must move his or her force in a consistent movement pattern in order to ensure accuracy. To establish accuracy and consistency in the swing, approach, and delivery, everything must move in straight lines toward the designated target.

The swing must stay in a straight forward and backward arc. Holding the ball off to the right side while in the stance will assure that it will travel in this straight line instead of moving in a circular pattern around the hips. Stabilizing the shoulders and wrist in the swing will also assist in keeping the swing straight.

The approach must be in a fairly straight line while moving toward the designated target. The shoulders and hips should be perpendicular to this target line as the feet move in a straight line toward the target. If the upper body position is kept square to the target, the swing will also stay square to the target (Figure 4.4).

The 10 o'clock thumb position for right handers and 2 o'clock for left handers must remain constant throughout the swing. To maintain this position, the wrist must remain firm and the forearm must not rotate.

Upon the release of the ball, everything is still square to the intended line of aim: the shoulders, the hips, the swing, and the follow-through. To fulfill and control the square-to-square concept, the entire body must be in perfect balance (Figure 4.5).

Controlling the entire body in the approach and the swing will assure

FIGURE 4.4 Upon delivery, the entire body is square to the target.

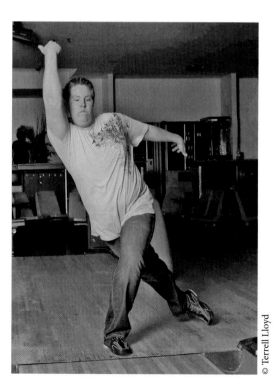

© Terrell Lloyd

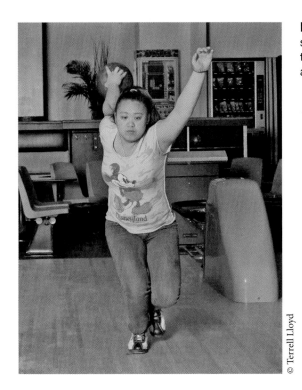

FIGURE 4.5 Keeping the shoulders and hips square to the target results in more accuracy.

© Terrell Lloyd

the bowler of rolling the ball the same way time after time. Once this consistency is conquered, the bowler can now start making accurate adjustments.

In summary, looking back upon Newton's Law of Motion, which states that an object at rest or in motion will remain at rest or in motion at the same speed, in a straight line, unless acted upon by an outside force, we find that every part of this law applies to bowling force production and accuracy. It is every bowler's object to control the variables in the skill of bowling in order to reach his or her potential. Once these variables are identified, error correction is also very easy.

References

Broer, Marion R. 1966. *Efficiency of human movement.* 2nd ed. Philadelphia: Saunders.

Culver, Elizabeth J. 1964. "Bowling." In Ainsworth, Dorothy S.: *Individual sports for women,* 4th ed. Philadelphia: Saunders.

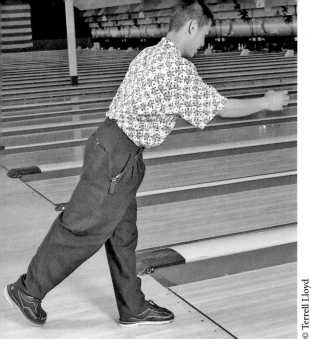

© Terrell Lloyd

5

Common Errors and Corrective Actions

The following chart of common bowling errors, effects, and corrective actions will assist a bowler or an instructor in developing diagnostic skills. However, due to the great number of movement variables and the interrelationship of these movements, it is impossible to cover every possible error and give the correct diagnosis for any particular individual's error. This chart is intended to assist the instructor in experiencing and sharpening diagnostic skills by analyzing the most common errors found in bowling. The concept of the error and corrections can more easily be identified by the cause-and-effect relationship as stated in the charts.

ERROR	CAUSE	EFFECT	CORRECTION
General:			
Lack of pin action	Lack of lift Lack of hook Lack of ball revolutions Ball rolls over thumb hole Lofting ball Overreaching Ball too light Late release Thumb hole too tight Improper pitches Ball line too far inside Ball line too far outside Skidding ball	Pins are left standing	Note: Check all corrections for these causes. Angle and proper revolutions are key to good pin action.
Backup ball (reverse hook)	Lack of knowledge of ball release and types of roll Thumb position at 12 o'clock and hand rotation Fingers in 6–7 o'clock position Starting with straight ball when learning to bowl Flexed wrist in stance or release Holding the ball in the middle of one's body Dropping right shoulder	Maximum ball deflection Lack of lift due to hyperextended wrist rotation Lack of consistency	Correct starting position (lining up shoulder with arrow). Hold ball in 8 or 9 o'clock position in stance. Firm wrist by pressing down with two outside fingers. Hold ball with forearm resting on hip in stance. Flex knees.
Stance:			
Feet too far apart	Attempt at body balance	Drifting Waddling	Move feet closer together.
Improper distribution of weight	Attempt at body balance	Not starting automatically with proper foot	Place most of the weight on balance-side foot.
Stiff knees	Bending too much at waist or leaning too far back	Large, awkward steps or not shuffling	Flex both knees equally.
Excessive forward body angle	Bending too much at waist	Stiff knees Loss of balance Tendency to rush	Straighten body enough to restore correct balance line.
Ball held too high	Ball held too high trying to get speed Slight aiming over ball	Release balance hand too soon Pushaway too long Steps too long Excessive approach speed High backswing	Establish ball height that will give smooth, controlled pendulum swing and desired speed.
Ball held too low	Excessive bending at waist	Push directly away too much Carrying ball during first step Timing off—body ahead of ball disrupts pendulum swing	Raise ball to desired height.
One heel up	One stiff knee	Balance and weight overshifted	Flex both knees equally.

ERROR	CAUSE	EFFECT	CORRECTION
Ball held in center of body	Ball feels comfortable equally supported with both hands	Tendency to hold thumb at 12 o'clock Tendency to flex wrist Tendency to develop outside-in arm swing or wrap-around swing Tendency to develop drift to left	Move ball position in line with right shoulders.
Elbow not tucked in	Elbow not tucked in to hip in stance Holding ball in center of body	Outside-in or wrap-around swing Incorrect and changing thumb position in swing	Place forearm on hip bone.
Wrist bent (Gooseneck)	Not enough pressure with index and little finger Loose grip Incorrect span	Ball slides too much and deflects Inconsistent delivery Painful knuckles	Press firmly against ball with two outside fingers or give support to wrist.
Wrist cupped	Overly firm wrist muscle flex	Locked elbow and shoulder, prohibiting natural pendulum swing and release Inconsistent delivery Restricted backswing	Relax arm and let ball drop naturally. Feel ball weight on fingers in stance.
Improper spread of outside fingers	Outside fingers either spread or close to middle fingers Lack of understanding of the effects of spread of either or both index or little finger	Not achieving maximum hooking/hitting potential	Hold outside fingers close if little or no turn desired. Spread index finger for semi-roller, if extra turn desired. Spread little finger for full-roller, if extra turn desired.
Weak grip	Not enough pressure exerted with two middle fingers Not enough pressure with two outside fingers Short span and/or large holes	Too much fluctuation of hand during swing Dropped ball Lack of backswing No lift	Put tension in wrist and fingers. Select ball with proper span and hole sizes.
Lack of concentration	Lack of confidence Distraction on approach Wandering mind Eyes not focused on target Self-induced pressure	Imperfect execution of delivery Carry-over frustration Low scores Inconsistent approach method	Develop simple, relaxed concentration—not grim, lip-biting, teeth-gritting determination.
Lack of relaxation	Grim determination Giving in to pressure of occasion Gripping ball too tightly Lack of proper breathing	Ball steered, pushed, or pulled in delivery Inability to sustain string of strikes	Take a deep breath—exhale. Flex knees. Loosen grip slightly. Feel looseness in elbow. Lean forward slightly, ready for smooth pushaway step.

ERROR	CAUSE	EFFECT	CORRECTION
Pushaway (First Step):			
Ball pushed too high	Attempt to develop speed Ball pushed up more than out Weight is back Ball is too light	Abrupt lowering of ball Low or high backswing Jerky swing Dropped shoulder Poor timing—bowler ahead of ball	Push ball in a downward direction.
Ball lowered too soon (little or no pushaway)	Ball pushed down more than out Attempt to get ball in backswing, quickly Leaning forward in stance Ball too heavy	Muscling the swing Ball not in the appropriate position at conclusion of first step Poor timing—ball is ahead of bowler	Push ball in a downward direction. Check ball weight. Push ball in outward direction. Extend elbows during pushaway.
Pushaway too long	Attempt to straighten arm and extend to full length for full pendulum swing	Step too long Feeling of rushing	Push ball a moderate distance forward and downward. Delay straightening of elbow. Avoid leaning forward with pushaway.
Ball pushed too far right or left	Try to clear the hip Lack of kinesthetic awareness	Developing inside-out or outside-in swing Missing target Dropping shoulder	Hold ball to side of body in front of shoulder and push ball toward target. Maintain thumb position created in stance.
Downswing (Second Step):			
Balance hand released too late	Not taking balance hand off ball Fear of dropping ball	Carrying ball Hurried downswing Stiff approach	The balance hand should be disengaged just as the first step is completed.
Left hand released too early (Figure 5.1)	Taking balance hand off ball too early	Muscling Hurried swing Dropped shoulder	The balance hand should be disengaged, just as the first step is completed.

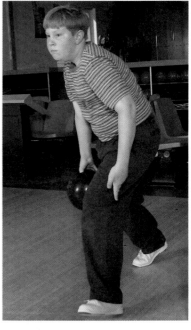

FIGURE 5.1   Release of left hand too soon in downswing.

ERROR	CAUSE	EFFECT	CORRECTION
Ball carried	Balance hand not disengaged Lack of pushaway Not using force of gravity	Timing off Inconsistent ball speed	Move ball first, let feet follow. Balance hand should be disengaged. Let gravitational force act upon the ball.
Lack of counter-balance	Balance arm not allowed to attain counter-balance position	Dropped shoulder	Simultaneously with the downward motion of the ball, extend the balance arm to the side of, and slightly away from, body.
Backswing (Third Step):			
Backswing too high (Figure 5.2)	Ball too light Pushaway too high and too forceful Attempt to get speed by deliberately raising ball in backswing Shoulder and hip allowed to tilt forward and rotate	Shoulder/hip rotation Possible sideways finish on fourth step Sidearming delivery Too much speed	Increase weight of ball. Control pushaway—let natural pendulum swing develop. Do not add speed in swing by "muscling." Flex knees and avoid bending at the waist.
Backswing too low	Inhibited swing Cupped wrist Muscling Ball too heavy	Muscling Forced release Early turn	Develop free pendulum swing. Push the ball slightly higher in pushaway. Decrease weight of ball.

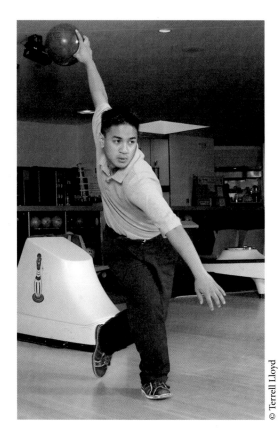

© Terrell Lloyd

FIGURE 5.2   Backswing too high.

ERROR	CAUSE	EFFECT	CORRECTION
Backswing (Third Step):			
Shoulder and hip rotation	Pushaway too forceful Attempt to get speed by deliberately increasing backswing	May result in sideways finish in fourth step Sidearming delivery	Control pushaway—develop free pendulum swing. Do not add speed to swing by "muscling." Maintain consistent thumb position. Maintain firm wrist throughout swing.
Hesitation at top of backswing	Bending too far forward Weight on toes Hunching shoulders	Inhibited fluid motion of swing Forced downswing	Restore body balance on balance line. Develop free pendulum swing.
Wrap-around swing	Ball held in center of body in stance Ball held to right of shoulders in stance Ball pushed to right during first step	Inconsistent ball path and direction	Keep shoulders square to target. Position ball in line with shoulder and push straight ahead.
Elbow bent	Over-controlling the ball Incorrect span	Inconsistent speed and delivery Sidearm release Lack of pendular swing	Extend elbow in pushaway. Feel gravitational pull of ball in downswing.
Swing "bumps" outward	Ball pushed away toward left	Misdirected follow-through Backup ball delivery Misdirected follow-through	Push toward target.
Wrist rotates inward	Shoulders not square to target and elbow out	Maintain hand and wrist position.	Keep shoulders square to target and elbow straight
Bowling shoulder dropped	Balance arm too high	Loss of balance to ball side	Maintain balance arm below shoulder level.
Timing (Fourth Step):			
Body ahead of ball	Sliding too far Lack of synchronized movement Lack of balance line Pushaway started late	Body balance lost Hurried released Dropped ball Pushed or pulled ball Sidearming in delivery	Bring ball forward with slide. Restore balance line. Slide only as far as body balance can be maintained. Move the ball first in pushaway.
Not enough slide	Stance too close to foul line Heel-toe approach Lack of balance line Picking up sliding foot Landing heel first Lack of flex in sliding knee	Crowded steps Abrupt stop Abrupt release Difficulty completing follow-through	Move stance further back. Shuffle during delivery. Develop balance line. Concentrate on sliding last step. Keep ball-side foot down longer before raising for balance.
Too much slide	Stance too far from foul line Overemphasis on slide Lack of balance line Right hip and shoulder remaining back Approach too fast	Too much space for steps Right hip and shoulder remaining back Improper lift on ball Poor balance line	Move stance closer to foul line. Maintain balance line during slide. Decrease speed of steps and flex knees.

ERROR	CAUSE	EFFECT	CORRECTION
Sliding on wrong foot (Photo 5.3)	Start approach on wrong foot Timing of steps and swing off	No follow-through, off balance Lack of accuracy and consistency	Place most weight on balance-side foot in stance. Practice coordination of steps and swing.
Hop or skip steps	Straightening sliding-side knee, heel comes in contact with approach too soon Ball at top of backswing too soon Poor timing	Erratic release Loss of balance	Restore balance line. Start pushaway later. Extend pushaway further out.
Sliding sideways (Figure 5.4)	Approach too fast Insufficient sliding Lack of knee bend Starting approach too close to foul line Trail leg in open position (not pigeon-toed)	Inconsistent release Dropped ball Improper lift on ball Swinging ball around	Decrease speed of steps and flex knees. Flex sliding knee. Keep trail leg pigeon-toed and in contact with floor.
Off-balance sideways (Figure 5.5)	Drifting on last step Lacking of counter balance Dropped shoulder Trail leg not counter-balancing	Pulling the ball off target Dropped shoulder Inconsistent release point— lofting or dropping Loses balance	Restore balance line. Develop and maintain counter-balance. Slide straight. Flex sliding knee. Keep trail leg as counter-balance to ball-side.

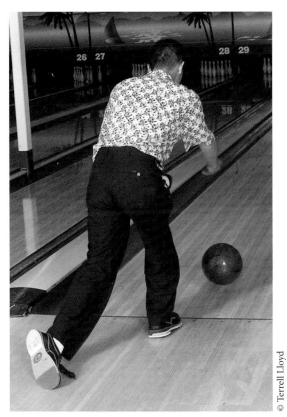

FIGURE 5.3   Sliding on the wrong foot.

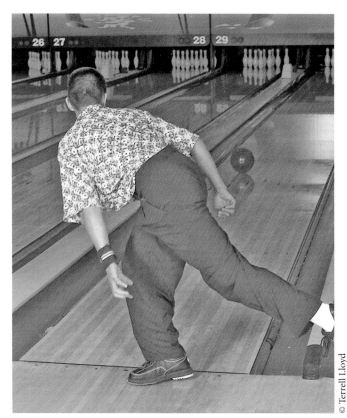

FIGURE 5.4   Foot turned sideways at the line.

ERROR	CAUSE	EFFECT	CORRECTION

Off-balance forward	Bending too much at waist
	Overreaching
	Steering or guiding ball
	Lunging
		Steering or guiding ball
		Lunging
		Lack of lift
		Late thumb release
			Restore balance line.
			Extending arm only enough
			  to complete pendulum
			  swing.
			Flex knees.
			Hold shoulders more
			  upright.
			Avoid kicking trail leg up
			  in air.

Rearing up	Attempt to achieve lift
	Attempt to get pin action
	Insecure thumb grip
		Loft of ball
		Muscled delivery
		Feel of "losing" ball
			Let momentum of ball
			  work.
			Check size of thumb hole
			  in downswing.
			Maintain knee bend and
			  balance line at release.
			Follow-through with arm,
			  not body.

Fouling (Figure 5.6)	Starting position too close
	Pushaway too long causing
	  steps to be too long
	Excessive slide
	Weight back on delivery
	Excessive approach speed
		Loss of pinfall on delivery	Control pushaway.
			If necessary, move back
			  approximately 6 inches at
			  a time to reestablish point of
			  origin.
			Establish balance line.
			Slow approach tempo.

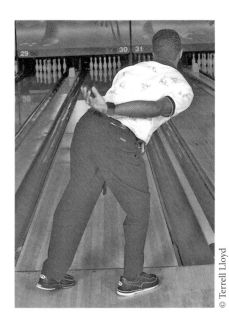

© Terrell Lloyd

FIGURE 5.5 Falling off the balance line.

FIGURE 5.6 Going over the foul line.

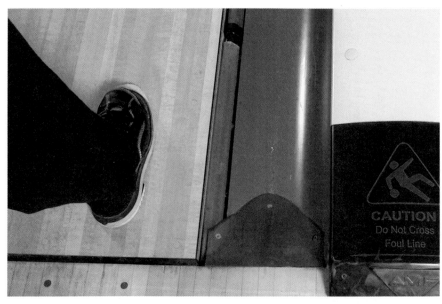

© Terrell Lloyd

ERROR	CAUSE	EFFECT	CORRECTION
Side-arming	Ball held in middle of body Inside-out or outside-in swing Attempting to "hook" ball	Inconsistent ball path Too much hook Missing target	Position ball in line with right shoulder. Control pushaway. Walk and slide straight to target. Keep elbow close to body during entire swing.
Ball released too soon	Body too straight on release Anxious to put "stuff" on ball Muscling downward Bent too far forward Stiff knee Ball held too loosely Finishing position too high or too low Incorrect ball fit	Lack of lift Ball hooks too much or not enough hook	Maintain natural pendulum swing. Restore balance line. Keep firm grip with all fingers. Restore balance line. Select ball with proper span and hole sizes. Snug thumb hole.
Ball released too late	Overreaching Steering (guiding) ball Thumb hole too tight Too much pitch in thumb hole Attempt to get "lift"	Steering (guiding) ball Skidding Inconsistent ball path Weak ball—no hitting power Loft	Maintain pendulum swing. Make sure thumb hole size and pitch allows free thumb release. Restore balance line. Grip ball firmly but without tension.
Release:			
Cut-off armswing (bent elbow) (Figure 5.7)	Not extending arm forward Eagerness to apply lift Using forearm too much Improper fit of ball Span too long	Inconsistent ball path and direction Lofting ball	Maintain pendulum swing. Firmness of grip plus pendulum swing will produce desired lift and roll. Maintain straight elbow on follow-through.
Dropped ball	Poor timing Throwing ball into approach or lane Too much weight on ball-side foot Holes too large and/or improper pitches Lack of balance line Incorrect span	Inconsistent ball path and direction	Synchronize movements. Restore balance line. Keep firm grip with all fingers. Hole sizes and pitches should allow ball control to be maintained until released beyond the bottom of pendulum arc. Select ball with the proper span.
Lofted ball	Stiff sliding-side knee Hanging on to ball too long Holes too small and/or too much pitch Attempt to get "lift"	Inconsistent ball path Ball skids too much, little roll or hook	Restore balance line. Maintain pendulum swing. Flex sliding-side knee. Check holes for size and pitch, especially thumb hole. Use less "muscle" at release point.

ERROR	CAUSE	EFFECT	CORRECTION
Not consistent in alignment and height of arm follow-through (Figure 5.8)	Poor timing Lack of balance line Faulty release Overreaching Exaggerated follow-through (Statue of Liberty) Forced completion of pendulum arc	Forced completion of pendulum arc Ball path and direction inconsistent execution	Synchronize movements. Restore balance line. Check release. Allow follow-through to be natural continuation of pendulum arc. Follow-through arm directly in front of shoulder.
Overall Delivery:			
Too fast	Ball held too high Pushaway too forceful Pushaway too long		Position ball in stance to encourage controlled pushaway and pendulum swing.
	Swing too fast Approach too long Bent too far forward	Poor timing Too much speed on ball Lack of hook Ball deflects	Decrease size of steps. Develop balance line.
Too slow	Standing too upright Uncertainty Carrying ball Approach too short Pushaway downward	Inconsistent release Too much hook Insufficient speed on ball	Develop pendulum swing. Let swing govern feet. Move point of origin back slightly. Push the ball out in a downward direction and accentuate the pushaway.

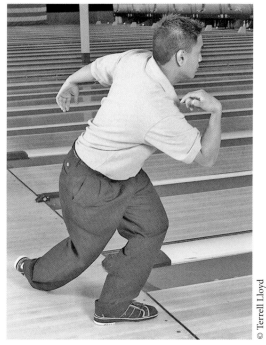

FIGURE 5.7 Short follow-through, early elbow flex.

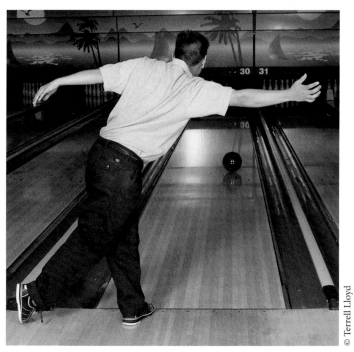

FIGURE 5.8 Sideways follow-through.

© Terrell Lloyd

ERROR	CAUSE	EFFECT	CORRECTION
Steps too long	Exaggerated pushaway	Approach looks and feels awkward Lack of fluid motion	Shorten steps—synchronize with pendulum swing.
Steps too short	Carrying ball Ball not pushed forward enough Letting footwork govern swing	Poor timing Approach looks and feels awkward Lack of fluid motion	Develop smooth controlled pushaway. Let pushaway and pendulum swing govern feet.
Ball "double-dribbled" at release	Excessive waist bend	Loss of ball action	Maintain balance line and direction at release. Check knee bend.
Ball rolling over holes	Poor wrist and finger position	Loss of roll and hook	Check fit of ball. Maintain firm wrist and finger position at release. Keep elbow firm during swing.
Drifting	Not aligned properly with target Feeling of too far right or left at point of origin Facing target incorrectly Pushing ball outside or inside shoulder line First step a cross-over or side-step Outside-in or inside-out swing Side-arming in delivery Misdirected follow-through Not keeping eyes on target	Develop outside-in or inside-out arm swing Side-arming in delivery Push or pull ball at release Looking at pins to see results	Align ball, shoulder, and target. Push ball straight ahead toward target. Step forward straight ahead. Maintain pendulum swing. Concentrate on target until ball passes over it.
Ball Path and Direction:			
Not enough hook	Too much speed Poor timing Overreaching Pushing Steering (guiding) ball Dropping ball Lofting Incorrect hand position Lack of lift Thumb hole too tight Overturn in release Skidding ball Ball too heavy Poor adjustment to lane conditions	Lack of hitting power Lack of proper angle of entry into pocket Maximizing deflection Ball travels through too much oil	Synchronize movements. Maintain pendulum swing. Keep firm wrist and finger grip. Keep fingers at 4-5 o'clock position throughout swing (generally). Check ball for weight and hook dynamics. Let thumb out of ball first and allow fingers to lift. Decrease approach and ball speed. Use a bowling ball with a duller, more porous surface. Adjust stance and target to the right. Adjust stance and target to the right.

ERROR	CAUSE	EFFECT	CORRECTION
Too much hook	Poor timing Pulling Insufficient ball speed Ball too light Early release Ball rolls too early Outside fingers too far on side of ball Excessive lift and/or excessive turn Poor adjustment to lane conditions	Ball rolls too early Lack of accuracy Depending upon the weight of ball—too much angle or too much deflection Ball traveling across dry portion of the lane	Synchronize movements. Maintain pendulum swing. Check firmness of grip and wrist not cupped. Check ball for hook dynamics. Lift through ball not acutely counter-clockwise. Adjust stance and target to the left. Use a bowling ball with shinier, less porous surface.
Inconsistent hook	Hand and wrist positions vary during approaches	Inability to roll ball across target Inconsistent impact points	Maintain firm wrist. Maintain consistent finger position. Deliver ball at same speed every time.
Ball generally too light in pocket	Excessive speed in delivery Ball line too deep Ball line too far outside Overreaching Pushing-steering ball Lack of lift Rearing Skidding ball Inside-out swing Wrap-around swing High backswing Drifting	Lack of striking power Maximum deflection	Control pushaway and maintain pendulum swing. Check starting and finishing position of slide foot to see if delivery foot steps are straight. Check thumb and finger position at release point. Maintain firm grip with wrist and fingers. Check balance line at release. Check position of ball in stance. Increase lift. Adjust starting position and target to the right.
Ball generally too heavy in pocket	Slow ball Ball line too deep Ball line too far outside Pulling ball Rearing Early release Excessive lift Outside-in swing Wrap-around swing Drifting	Excessive split and spare leaves Acute angle of entry	Check starting and finishing position of slide foot to see if delivery foot steps are straight. Control pushaway and maintain pendulum swing. Check thumb and finger position at release point. Maintain firm grip with wrist and fingers. Check balance line at release. Check position of ball in stance. Follow-through in line with shoulder. Avoid rearing up. Check the arm position in stance and direction of pushaway. Adjust starting position and target to the left.

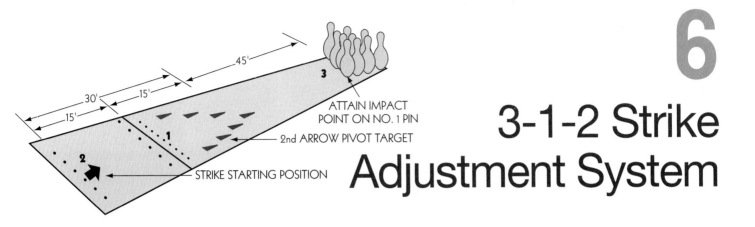

45'

30'

15'

15'

3

ATTAIN IMPACT
POINT ON NO. 1 PIN

1

2nd ARROW PIVOT TARGET

2

STRIKE STARTING POSITION

6

3-1-2 Strike Adjustment System

One of the more challenging aspects of the bowling game is adjusting to changing **lane conditions.** Even lanes within the same establishment play differently due to atmospheric conditions, time of day, the quality and amount of play, or the difference in maintenance procedures. Because of these differences in characteristics, the bowling ball may hook more or less from one lane to another. It is the bowler's responsibility to adjust to the lane. As long as the bowler can reasonably deliver the ball consistently in the same way, adjustments can be made.

The **3-1-2 strike adjustment system,** the most fundamental adjustment in bowling, is based on a mathematical computation that will aid in determining how much delivery adjustment is needed. It takes the guesswork out of adjusting the strike-ball delivery, but it only applies to the first delivery of a frame.

The adjustment takes place in the delivery stance after judging where the ball is consistently contacting the pins in relation to the head pin. Remember, the second target arrow remains the constant point of aim. The

only thing that should be adjusted is the foot position in a new point of origin. The **basic rule of thumb** is to move in the direction of the error or mistake. If you deliver the ball and the ball hooks too much, traveling left of the 17th board, move the stance left. If the ball goes too far right, move right.

Before going any further, a quick review is needed.

For Right Handers

- The head pin is on the 20th board.
- The 1-3 pocket is on the 17th board.
- The 3 pin is near the 14th board.
- The Brooklyn pocket is near the 23rd board (Figure 6.1).

For Left Handers

- The head pin is on the 20th board.
- The 1-2 strike pocket is on the 17th board from the left.
- The 3 pin is on the 26th board from the left.
- The crossover pocket of the 1-3 is near the 23rd board from the left (Figure 6.2).

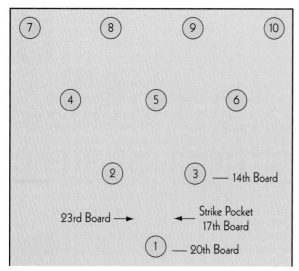

FIGURE 6.1 (Right Handers) Pins and corresponding boards.

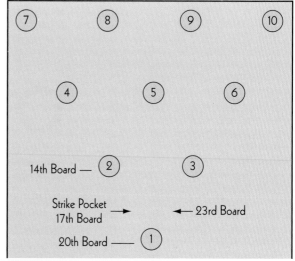

FIGURE 6.2 (Left Handers) Pins and corresponding boards.

With the previous information in mind, the bowler can make adjustments by determining the number of boards separating the pocket from the actual point of contact of the ball. Specifically, this 3-1-2 system states, **for every 3 boards the ball is off at the pins, move the feet in the stance 2 boards in the direction of the error** (Figures 6.3 and 6.4).

For Right Handers

If the ball is properly delivered and rolls over the second arrow but strikes the head-pin flush, leaving big splits time after time, the following adjustment should be made. Knowing the head pin is on the 20th board and the 1-3 pocket is on the 17th board, the bowler is able to determine that this ball roll is 3 boards left of the pocket. Using the 3-1-2 formula, move the stance 2 boards to the left (Figure 6.5).

On another day or lane, the ball may be consistently entering the Brooklyn pocket. The Brooklyn pocket is 6 boards to the left of the 1-3 pocket, so the needed adjustment to be made is moving the point of origin 4 boards to the left (Figure 6.6).

And on yet another day or lane, the ball may roll down the lane and contact the 3-pin flush, missing the head pin altogether. The 3 pin is approximately 3 boards away from the pocket, so the adjustment is made by moving the point of origin 2 boards to the right (Figure 6.7).

For Left Handers

If the ball is properly delivered and rolls over the second arrow from the left but strikes the head-pin flush, leaving big splits time after time, the following adjustment should be made. Knowing the head pin is on the 20th board and the 1-2 pocket (strike pocket for left handers) is on the 17th board from the left, the bowler is able to determine that this ball roll is 3 boards right of the pocket. Using the 3-1-2 formula, move the stance 2 boards to the right of your original point of origin (Figure 6.8).

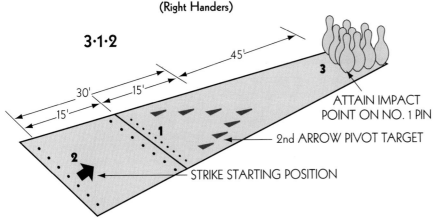

STRIKE ADJUSTMENT SYSTEM
(Right Handers)

3·1·2

45'

30'

15'

15'

3

ATTAIN IMPACT POINT ON NO. 1 PIN

1

2nd ARROW PIVOT TARGET

1

2

STRIKE STARTING POSITION

FIGURE 6.3
The 3-1-2 Strike Adjustment System for right-handers. (Courtesy of former NBC)

FIGURE 6.4   The 3-1-2 Strike Adjustment System for left-handers. (Courtesy of former NBC)

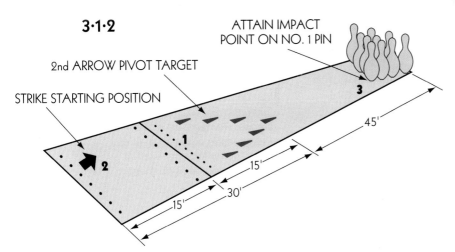

STRIKE ADJUSTMENT SYSTEM
(Left Handers)

3·1·2

ATTAIN IMPACT POINT ON NO. 1 PIN

2nd ARROW PIVOT TARGET

STRIKE STARTING POSITION

3

1

2

45'

15'

30'

15'

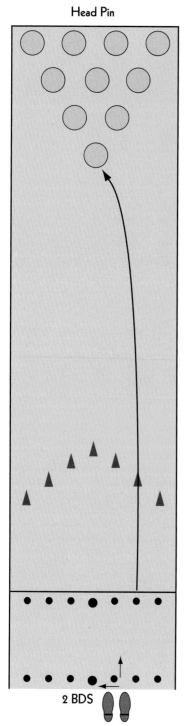

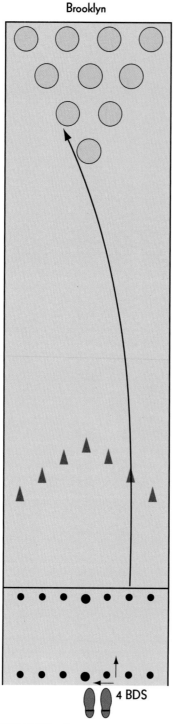

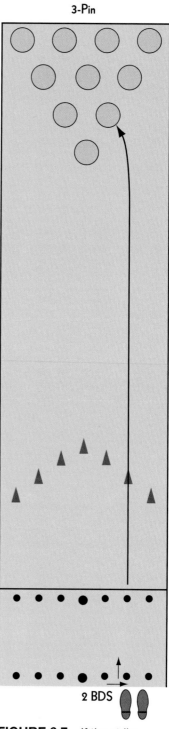

FIGURE 6.5 (Right-hand adjustments). If the strike ball consistently hits the head-pin flush, move feet *2 boards left in stance.*

FIGURE 6.6 If the strike ball consistently hits the Brooklyn pocket (1-2 pins), move feet *4 boards left in stance.*

FIGURE 6.7 If the strike ball consistently hits the 3-pin flush, move *2 boards right in stance.* **Remember:** Move in the direction of the error. (If ball goes too far left, move left. If ball goes too far right, move right.)

Head Pin

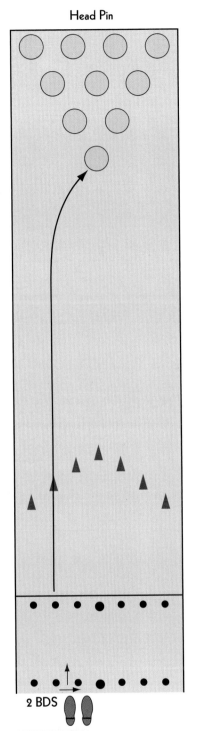

Brooklyn

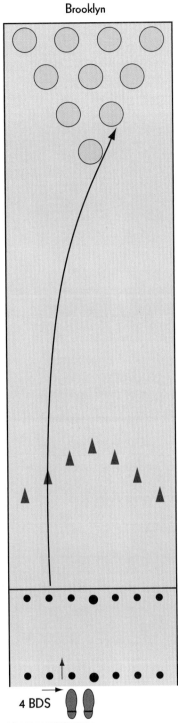

2-Pin

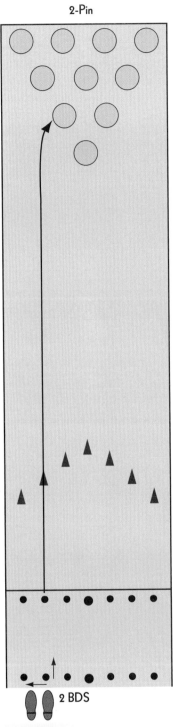

FIGURE 6.8   (Left-hand adjustments). If the strike ball consistently hits the head-pin flush, move *2 boards right in stance.*

FIGURE 6.9   If the strike ball consistently crosses over to the Brooklyn pocket (1-3 pins), move *4 boards right in stance.*

FIGURE 6.10   If the strike ball consistently hits the 2-pin flush, move *2 boards left in stance.*

On another day or lane, the ball may be consistently entering the crossover 1-3 pocket. This pocket is 6 boards to the right of the 1-2 pocket, so the needed adjustment would be to move the point of origin 4 boards to the right (Figure 6.9). And yet, on another day or lane, the ball may roll down the lane and contact the 2-pin flush, missing the head pin altogether. The 2 pin is approximately 3 boards left of the 1-2 pocket, so the adjustment is made by moving the point of origin 2 boards to the left (Figure 6.10).

This adjustment system will work only when the bowler faces and walks toward the target arrow. This will result in the bowler walking at a slight angle and playing the lane on diagonals. Walking toward the target arrow will put the bowler in the proper delivery position, and will prohibit the bowler from following through with poor direction or dropping the shoulder to hit the target.

Mathematical Formula

How does this system work mathematically? We have already established that it is 75 feet from the third row of locator dots to the head pin. The distance from the starting position to the target arrow (the pivot point) is approximately 30 feet. That leaves a 45-foot spread from the target arrow to the head pin, so the ball has another 15 feet farther to roll. Putting this into a ratio, the stance-to-target ratio is 30 feet to 75 feet, with the target pin ratio at 45 feet to 75 feet. Breaking into smaller fractions, it is a ratio of two-fifths to three-fifths, or 2:3. If the bowler makes a 2-board adjustment in the starting position, and the ball rolls across the same target arrow, the result is a 3-board change when the ball hits

the pins. This is all due to the length of the lane involved and the distance between the starting position, the target, and the pins.

Once the bowler makes an adjustment, it is necessary to turn the body and feet to face the target arrow and to walk toward it during the approach. This will result in a 1-board change (or adjustment) at the point of release at the foul line. It is 15 feet from the start to the foul line and another 15 feet from the foul line to the target. Thus, if the bowler, for example, adjusts 2 boards left in the stance, then the sliding foot at release point would actually be 1 board to the left of the old point of origin.

Words of Advice

When using this system, one must heed a few words of advice. Don't make adjustments on the basis of a single delivery or poor deliveries. Be certain that it was a good delivery and that it did go over the target arrow consistently. Don't confuse "pulling the ball" with too much hook; or following through toward the right with too little hook.

Additionally, keep in mind that this system works very well if making one or two adjustments (2- to 4-board adjustment in the stance, either left or right). However, if a third adjustment is attempted, the system tends to break down because, at this point, it becomes necessary to also make a target adjustment. Nevertheless, there should be no problem moving a total of 4 boards in either direction.

This system can also be used if the strike ball is hitting light (more on the 3 pin than the 1) or heavy (more on the 1 pin than the 3) by moving half the distance in the stance or 1 board. Again, this follows the formula because this means the ball is hitting the pocket at the 15.5 board and the

Self Evaluation QUESTIONS

1. After your foot adjustments in the 3-1-2, in what direction do you take your approach?

2. What stance adjustments must be made if the strike ball consistently hits the following?
   a. Head pin
   b. Heavy on the 3
   c. Heavy on the 1

18.5 board, respectively. The error is one-half of the 3 board error, or 1.5 off target. If the bowler uses a ratio of 3:2, the feet would be adjusted 1 board in the stance.

In a Nutshell:

- The 3-1-2 strike adjustment system is mathematically formulated according to the dimensions of the lane.
- For every 3 boards the ball is off when it hits the pins, move 2 boards in the starting position.
- Move the stance in the direction of the error or mistake. If the ball goes too far to the right, move right, or vice versa.
- With this stance, the body and feet must be square to the target, the intended line of ball roll, and *not* the foul line.
- When executed properly, the bowler's slide foot at release point should *not* be on the same board as aligned in the stance. The bowler should have intentionally "drifted" or walked toward the target.
- This system only works within a 4-board stance adjustment in either direction.
- This system works in any proportion of the mathematical ratio.

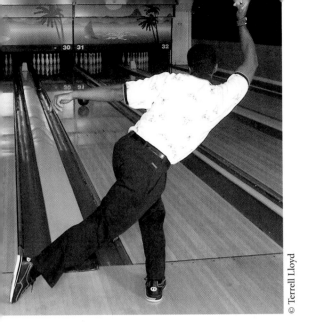
© Terrell Lloyd

7

3-6-9 Spare Conversion System

The 3-6-9 spare system is the most basic of all spare conversion systems. It has been scientifically developed for accuracy and uses a constant target for consistency and ease of learning. It is a system that takes the guesswork out of spare conversions.

Before this spare adjustment system can be implemented, the bowler must be cognizant of the following principles:

The key pin must be identified in all spare conversion attempts.

- If the key pin happens to be one of the strike ball or center of the lane pins, there is no, or very little, adjustment that takes place from the strike-ball delivery.
- The basic rule of thumb for pins remaining to the right or left of the center pins is to move the stance origin to the side of the approach area opposite the location of the pins standing (Figures 7.1 and 7.2). If the pins remain standing in the center of the lane, the strike-ball stance and target are used.

The adjustments to pick up pins to the left and right of center are made from two points of origin:

Right Handers:

- All adjustments for pins remaining on the left of center are made from the correct point of origin for the strike-ball delivery.
- All adjustments for pins remaining on the right of center are made from the correct point of origin for the 10-pin delivery.

Left Handers:

- All adjustments for pins remaining on the right of center are made from the correct point of origin for the strike-ball delivery.
- All adjustments for pins remaining on the left of center are made from the correct point of origin for the 7-pin delivery.

Key Pin Identification

The strike-ball point of origin has been established in the previous chapter, so now we need to learn how to locate the key pin. The key pin is the pin that needs to be contacted for all other pins to fall. It is the only pin on which to focus attention during a

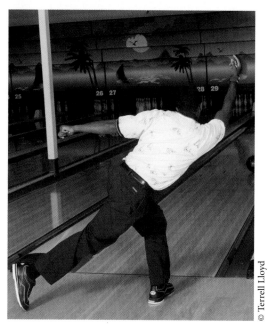

FIGURE 7.1 A right hander converting a 7 pin.

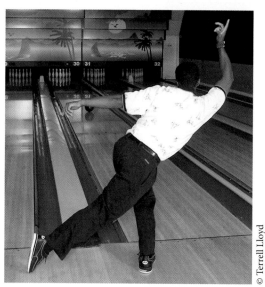

FIGURE 7.2 A right hander converting a 10 pin.

© Terrell Lloyd

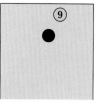

Key pin in 2-pin leave

Key pin in 3-pin leave

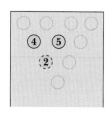

Key pin in baby 4–5 split

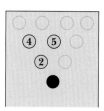

Key pin in 4-pin leave with headpin

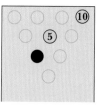

Key pin in splits other than baby splits

FIGURE 7.3 A-E Key pins for basic spare conversion.

spare conversion. This pin in a 2-pin leave is the closest to the bowler (Figure 7.3A). In a 3-pin cluster, it is the pin in the middle (Figure 7.3B). In a baby split (where the ball can be fitted in between the two pins), it is the pin missing between the 2 pins left standing (Figure 7.3C). If four or more pins are standing and the head pin is one of them, the head pin is the key pin (Figure 7.3D). In a split where the pins are greater than 12 inches apart, the key pin is the pin, either real or imaginary, adjacent to the one closest to you on the outside of the combination (Figure 7.3E).

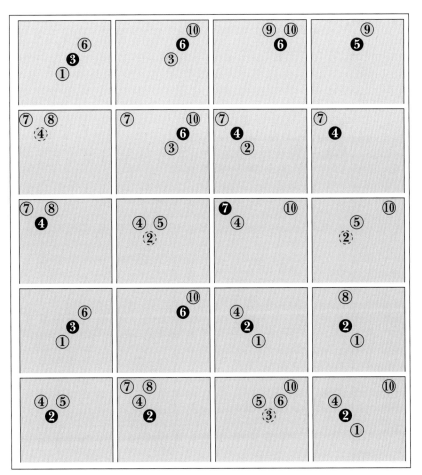

FIGURE 7.4   Identifying the key pin.

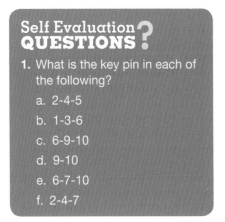

Right Hander's 3-6-9 Spare Conversion System for Converting Pins Left of Center

In converting pins to the left of the head pin, the key pin must be located and then, using the rule of thumb, the feet will be moved right of the strike-ball origin (Figures 7.5, 7.6A, and 7.6B). For each pin to the left of the head pin, the feet will be moved right 3 boards while going over the second arrow from the right. To convert the 2 pin, or any combination of the 2 pin (2-4-5, 2-8, 1-2-4, and so on),

move the starting stance 3 boards to the right of the strike-ball stance, aim for the second target arrow from the right, and walk toward the 2 pin slightly (Figures 7.7A and 7.7B). The 2 pin, or any combination involving the 2 pin, will be covered by the ball, providing the delivery is consistent. To convert the 4 pin, or any 4-pin combination, the bowler must move 6 boards to the right of the strike ball stance, aim for the same second target arrow, and walk toward the 4 pin (Figures 7.8A and 7.8B).

When the 7 pin is left standing, or when it is the key pin, the bowler will move 9 boards to the right of the strike-ball stance, aim for the second arrow, and walk toward the pin (Figures 7.9A and 7.9B).

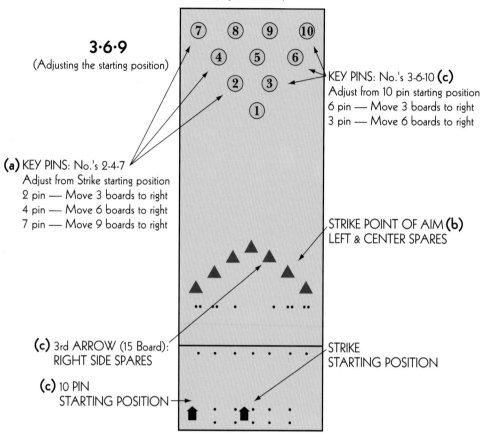

SPARE ADJUSTMENT SYSTEM
(Right Handers)

3·6·9
(Adjusting the starting position)

(a) KEY PINS: No.'s 2-4-7
Adjust from Strike starting position
2 pin — Move 3 boards to right
4 pin — Move 6 boards to right
7 pin — Move 9 boards to right

KEY PINS: No.'s 3-6-10 **(c)**
Adjust from 10 pin starting position
6 pin — Move 3 boards to right
3 pin — Move 6 boards to right

STRIKE POINT OF AIM **(b)**
LEFT & CENTER SPARES

(c) 3rd ARROW (15 Board):
RIGHT SIDE SPARES

STRIKE
STARTING POSITION

(c) 10 PIN
STARTING POSITION

FIGURE 7.5 Right-hander's Spare Adjustment System.
a. The 3-6-9 adjustment for left-side spares.
b. The spare angle and target arrow used for the 10 pin.
c. The 3-6 adjustment made for right-side spares.

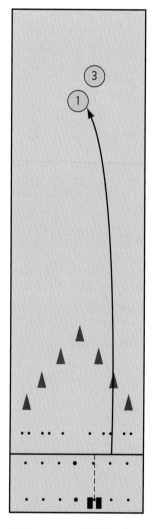

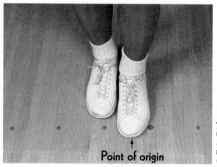

FIGURE 7.6A and 7.6B
Right-hander's strike point
of origin.

Point of origin

© Eric Risberg

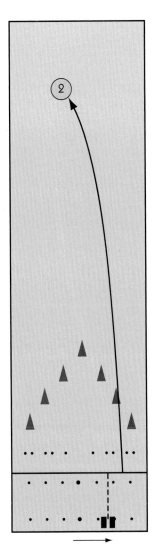

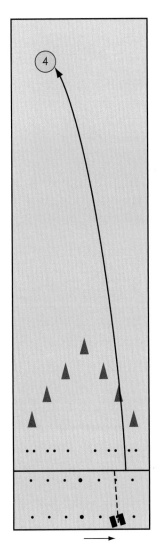

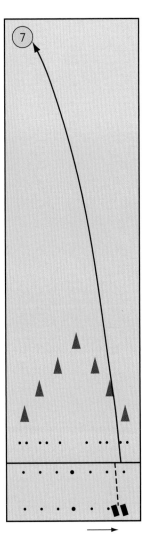

FIGURE 7.7A 2-Pin spare—Move 3 boards to the right from the strike-ball point of origin.

FIGURE 7.8A 4-Pin spare—Move 6 boards to the right from the strike-ball point of origin.

FIGURE 7.9A 7-Pin spare—Adjust 9 boards to the right from the strike-ball point of origin.

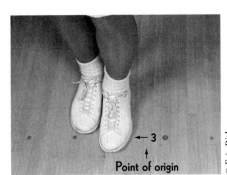

© Eric Risberg

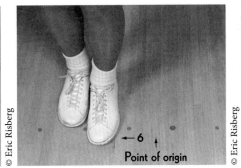

© Eric Risberg

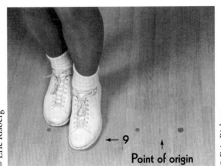

© Eric Risberg

FIGURE 7.7B 2-Pin spare—Adjust 3 boards to the right from the strike-ball point of origin.

FIGURE 7.8B 4-Pin spare—Adjust 6 boards to the right from the strike-ball point of origin.

FIGURE 7.9B 7-Pin spare—Adjust 9 boards to the right from the strike-ball point of origin.

Self Evaluation?
QUESTIONS?

1. What will your point of origin be to convert the following key pins?

a. 4 pin

b. 7 pin

c. 2 pin

d. 8 pin

e. 5 pin

Remember: If the bowler walks toward the key pin, it will put the body at a slight angle to the foul line. This is the only way these spare adjustments will work properly. The shoulders are square to the target arrow and the key pin not to the foul line.

The importance of delivering and rolling the ball the same way, over the same target arrow, changing the point of origin, cannot be overemphasized in the 3-6-9 system. This only changes the approach angle slightly and allows the conversion of spares without changing the arm swing or movement toward the foul line.

Right Hander's 3-6-9 Spare Conversion System for Converting Pins Right of Center

Conversion of right-side spares uses the same theory as just discussed; however, the point of origin and the target changes. Instead of using the strike-ball origin, one now adjusts from the 10-pin point of origin, always using the third target arrow from the right (Figure 7.5).

To find the point of origin for the 10 pin, the stance, using the left foot as a guide, should be at the place near the left edge of the lane at least 15

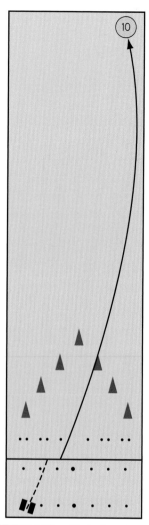

FIGURE 7.10A   Right-hander's 10-pin point of origin.

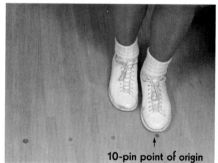

10-pin point of origin

© Eric Risberg

FIGURE 7.10B   Right-hander's 10-pin point of origin.

boards left of center (Figures 7.10A and 7.10B). Draw an imaginary line through the third arrow from the right to the 10 pin. Still on the left, walk toward the 10 pin and deliver the ball in the same place. If the ball

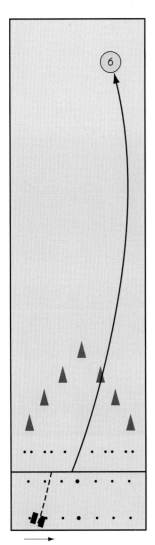

FIGURE 7.11A
6 Pin—Move 3 boards right of 10-pin point of origin.

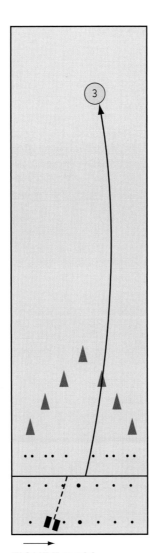

FIGURE 7.12A
3 Pin—Move 6 boards right of 10-pin point of origin.

goes into the channel, move a board or two to the right. If the ball goes too far to the left of the 10 pin, move a board or two to the left. When the correct adjustments have been made, and when it is certain the right origin board has been found for the 10 pin, the spare adjustments for the other pins on the right of center may be made. Again using the rule of thumb, for the right of center spares, find the key pin and then move 3 boards to the right of your 10-pin stance for each pin away from the 10 pin that the key pin is located. Go over the third arrow from the right.

To convert the 6 pin, or any combination of the 6 pin, move 3 boards right of the 10-pin origin point, face the third target arrow, walk and swing toward the 6 pin (Figures 7.11A and 7.11B). For the 3-pin conversion, or any combination of the 3 pin, move 6 boards to the right of the 10-pin point of origin, face the target arrow, walk and swing toward the 3 pin (Figures 7.12A and 7.12B).

A spare conversion involving the 1 pin or the 5 pin is the basic strike ball. No adjustment from your strike-ball point of origin or target is necessary.

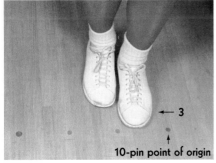

FIGURE 7.11B   6 Pin—Adjust 3 boards to the right from the 10-pin point of origin.

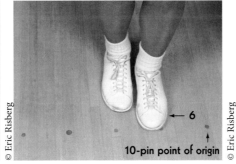

FIGURE 7.12B   3 Pin—Adjust 6 boards to the right from the 10-pin point of origin.

Self Evaluation QUESTIONS?

1. What will be your point of origin in order to convert the following key pins?
   a. 5 pin
   b. 6 pin
   c. 9 pin
   d. 10 pin
   e. 3 pin

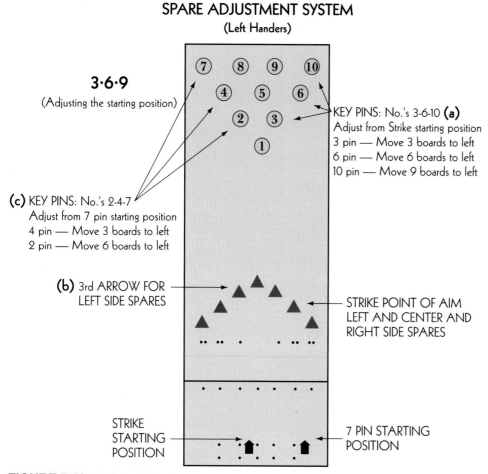

SPARE ADJUSTMENT SYSTEM
(Left Handers)

3·6·9
(Adjusting the starting position)

KEY PINS: No.'s 3-6-10 **(a)**
Adjust from Strike starting position
3 pin — Move 3 boards to left
6 pin — Move 6 boards to left
10 pin — Move 9 boards to left

(c) KEY PINS: No.'s 2-4-7
Adjust from 7 pin starting position
4 pin — Move 3 boards to left
2 pin — Move 6 boards to left

(b) 3rd ARROW FOR
LEFT SIDE SPARES

STRIKE POINT OF AIM
LEFT AND CENTER AND
RIGHT SIDE SPARES

STRIKE
STARTING
POSITION

7 PIN STARTING
POSITION

FIGURE 7.13   Left-hander's Spare Adjustment System.
a. 3-6-9 adjustment for the right-side spares.
b. The spare angle and target arrow for the 7 pin.
c. The 3-6 adjustment for left-side spares.

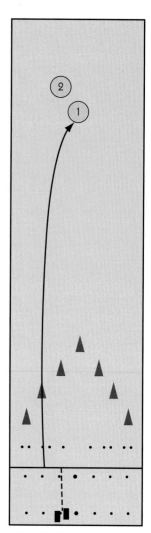

FIGURE 7.14A   Strike ball.

Left Hander's 3-6-9 Spare Conversion System for Converting Pins Right of Center

On spare conversions where the pins standing are right of the head pin, the key pin must be located and then, using the 3-6-9 rule of thumb, the feet will be moved left of the strike-ball origin (Figures 7.13, 7.14A, and 7.14B). For each pin to the right of the head pin, the feet will be moved left 3 boards while as far right-handers going over the second arrow from the left. To convert the 3 pin or any

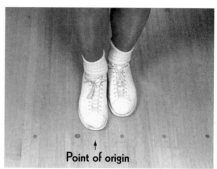

Point of origin

FIGURE 7.14B   Left-hander's strike point of origin.

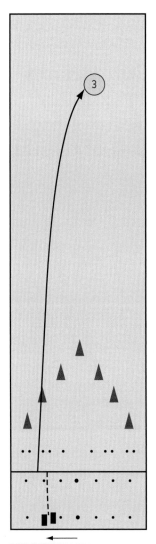

FIGURE 7.15A   3 Pin—Move 3 boards left of strike-ball point of origin.

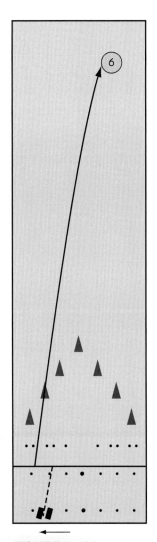

FIGURE 7.16A   6 Pin—Move 6 boards left of strike-ball point of origin.

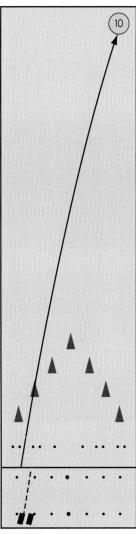

FIGURE 7.17A   10 Pin—Move 9 boards left of strike-ball point of origin.

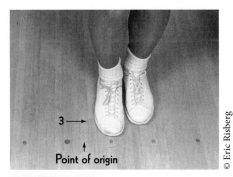

FIGURE 7.15B   3-Pin spare—Adjust 3 boards to the left from the strike-ball point of origin.

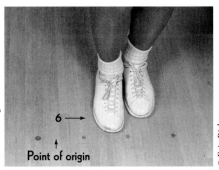

FIGURE 7.16B   6 Pin—Adjust 6 boards to the left from the strike-ball point of origin.

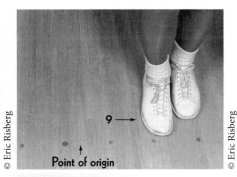

FIGURE 7.17B   10 Pin—Adjust 9 boards to the left from the strike-ball point of origin.

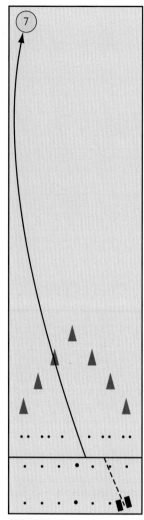

FIGURE 7.18A   7-Pin point of origin and third arrow.

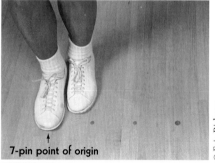

FIGURE 7.18B   Left-hander's 7-pin point of origin.

© Eric Risberg

combination of the 3 pin (3-5-10, 3-5-6, 1-3-6, 3-9, and so on), move the starting stance 3 boards to the left of your strike-ball stance, aiming for the second arrow from the left, and walking slightly toward the 3 pin (Figures 7.15A and 7.15B).

To convert the 6 pin or any 6-pin combination, the bowler must move 6 boards left of the strike-ball stance, aiming for the second arrow from the left, and walking toward the 6 pin (Figures 7.16A and 7.16B).

When the 10 pin is left standing, the bowler will move 9 boards left of the strike-ball stance, aim for the second arrow from the left, and walk toward the 10 pin (Figures 7.17A and 7.17B).

Self Evaluation QUESTIONS ?

1. Where will your point of origin be to convert the following key pins?

   a. 3 pin

   b. 10 pin

   c. 5 pin

   d. 9 pin

   e. 6 pin

Left Hander's 3-6-9 Spare Conversion System for Converting Pins Left of Center

Conversion of left-side spares uses the same theory as just discussed in the spare conversions right of center. However, the point of origin and the target change. Instead of using the strike ball point of origin, a left-handed bowler now adjusts from the 7-pin point of origin, always using the third arrow from the left as the target (Figure 7.13). To find the point of origin for the 7 pin, the stance, using the right foot as a guide, should be placed near the right edge of the lane, at least 15 boards right of center (Figures 7.18A and 7.18B). Draw an imaginary line through the third arrow from the left to the 7 pin that your ball would likely follow. Still on the right, walk toward the 7 pin and deliver the ball over the third arrow from the left. If the ball goes into the channel, move a board or two to the left. If the ball goes too far to the right of the 7 pin, move a board or two to the right. When the correct adjustments have been made, and when it is certain that the right origin board has been found for the 7 pin, the spare adjustments for the other pins left of center may be made.

Rule of thumb: For the left-of-center spares, find the key pin and move 3 boards left from the 7-pin stance for each pin away from the 7 pin that the key pin is located. Go over the third arrow from the left. To convert the 4 pin, or any combination involving the 4 pin, move 3 boards left of the 7-pin point of origin, face the third target arrow from the left,

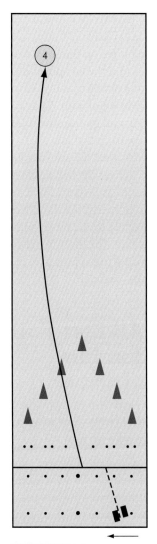

FIGURE 7.19A
4 Pin—Move 3 boards left
of 7-pin point of origin.

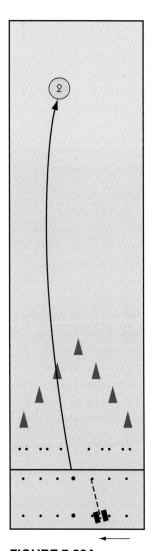

FIGURE 7.20A
2 Pin—Move 6 boards left
of 7-pin point of origin.

walk and swing toward the 4 pin
(Figures 7.19A and 7.19B). For the
2-pin conversion, or any combination
involving the 2 pin, move 6 boards
left of the 7-pin point of origin, face
the third arrow from the left, walk
and swing toward the 2 pin (Figures
7.20A and 7.20B). A spare conversion
involving the 1 or 5 pin is the basic
strike ball. No adjustment from your
strike ball stance is needed.

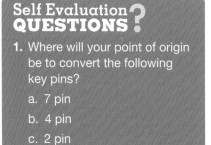

Self Evaluation?
QUESTIONS?

1. Where will your point of origin
be to convert the following
key pins?
a. 7 pin
b. 4 pin
c. 2 pin
d. 8 pin

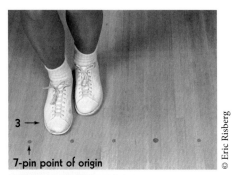

FIGURE 7.19B 4 Pin—Adjust
3 boards to the left from the 7-pin
point of origin.

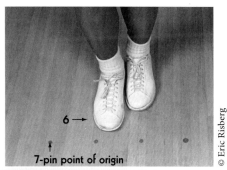

FIGURE 7.20B 2 Pin—Adjust 6
boards to the left from the 7-pin point
of origin.

In a Nutshell:

Using this 3-6-9 formula, spare conversions become simple and almost automatic. Remember these basic points while using the 3-6-9 adjustment system:

Right Handers:

- Locate the key pin.
- For spare leaves to the left of center, your point of aim is the second target arrow from the right. For spare leaves on the right, focus on the third target arrow from the right.
- For a leave to the left of center, adjust your starting position by moving 3, 6, or 9 boards to the right of your strike-ball point of origin. Do this in accordance with your key pin.
- For a leave on the right side of the lane, find the key pin and adjust to this pin by moving either 3 or 6 boards to the right of your 10-pin point of origin.
- Always walk toward the key pin and deliver the ball in the same manner as the strike ball. If delivered properly, the shoulders will be square to the target and not to the foul line. The footwork should be crossing the approach area at a slight diagonal.

Left Handers:

- Locate the key pin.
- For spare leaves to the right of center, your point of aim is the second target arrow from the left. For spare leaves to the left of center, your target arrow is the third arrow from the left.
- For a leave right of center, adjust your starting position by moving 3, 6, or 9 boards to the left of your strike-ball point of origin and go over your second board from the

left. Do this in accordance with your key pin.
- For a leave on the left side of the lane, find the key pin and adjust to this pin by moving either 3 or 6 boards left of your 7-pin point of origin and go over the third target arrow from the left.
- Always walk toward your key pin and deliver the ball in the same manner as the strike ball. If delivered properly, the shoulders will be square to the target and not the foul line. The footwork should be crossing the approach area at a slight diagonal.

"If All Else Fails" Addendum

Right Handers' Alternative Method of Converting Spares to the Right of Center

In the case where a bowler cannot grasp the above 3-6-9 method of converting spares that are to the right of center, an alternative method is being presented. Instead of making the adjustments from the 10-pin stance and going over the third arrow as previously stated in this chapter, try moving the stance to the left of your strike-ball stance 9, 12, or 15 boards while moving your target to the third arrow from the right. This would be your new formula:

To pick up the 3 pin or 9 pin, move 9 boards to the left of your strike-ball stance and go over the third arrow from the right (Figure 7.21A).

To pick up the 6 pin, move 12 boards to the left of your strike-ball stance and go over the third arrow from the right (Figure 7.21B).

To pick up the 10 pin, move 15 boards to the left of your strike-ball stance and go over the third arrow from the right (Figure 7.21C).

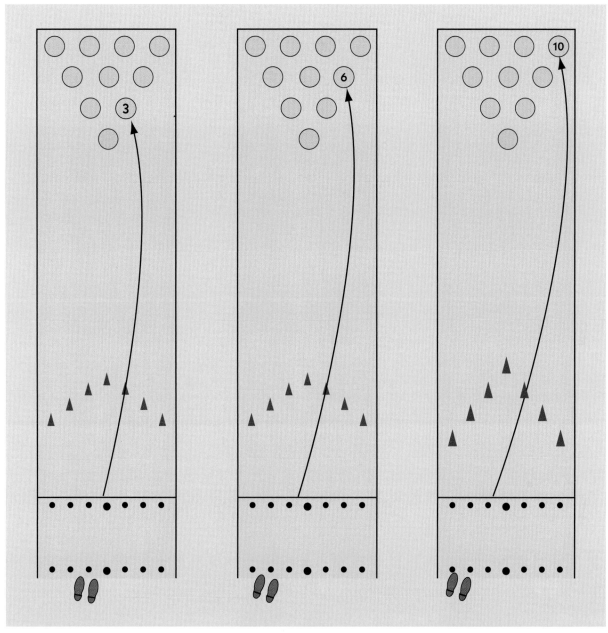

FIGURE 7.21A
3 Pin—Move 9 boards
left of strike-ball point of
origin—Use third arrow.

FIGURE 7.21B   6 Pin—
Move 12 boards left of
strike-ball point of origin—
Use third arrow.

FIGURE 7.21C
10 Pin—Move 15 boards
(3 dots) to left of strike-ball
point of origin—Use third
arrow.

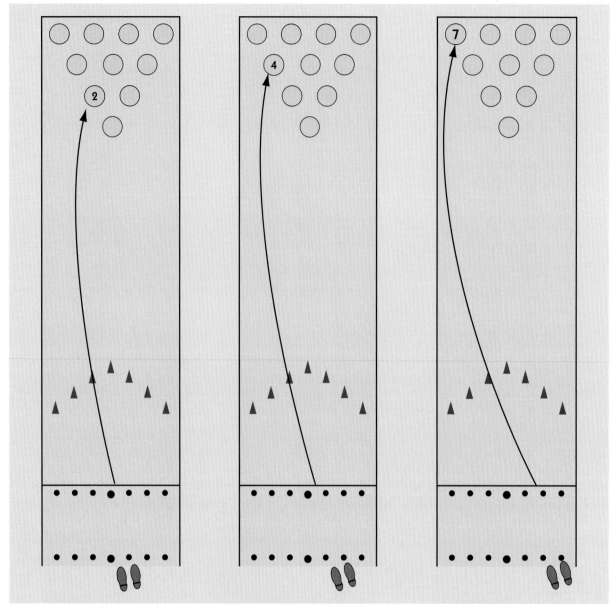

FIGURE 7.22A   2 Pin—Move 9 boards to right of strike-ball point of origin—Go over third arrow.

FIGURE 7.22B   4 Pin—Move 12 boards to right of strike-ball point of origin—Go over third arrow.

FIGURE 7.22C   7 Pin—Move 15 boards to the right of strike-ball point of origin—Go over third arrow.

Left Handers' Alternative Method of Converting Spares to the Left of Center

In the case where a bowler cannot grasp the above 3-6-9 method of converting spares that are to the left of center for left handers, an alternative method is being presented. Instead of making the adjustments from the 7-pin stance as previously stated in the chapter, try moving the stance to the right of your strike-ball 9-12 or 15 boards while moving your target to the third arrow from the left. This would be your new formula:

To pick up the 2 or 8 pin, move 9 boards to the right of your strike-ball stance and go over the third arrow from the left (Figure 7.22A). To pick up the 4 pin, move 12 boards to the right of your strike-ball stance and go over the third arrow from the right (Figure 7.22B).

To pick up the 7 pin, move 15 boards to the right of your strike-ball stance and go over the third arrow from the right (Figure 7.22C).

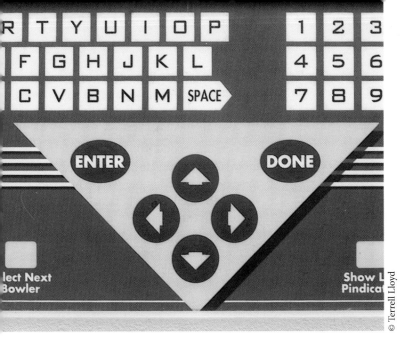

© Terrell Lloyd

8

Scoring and the Rules of Bowling

Scoring

It is a must that everyone who engages in the sport of bowling learn how to keep score and know the basic rules of the game. Yes, most modern bowling establishments now have automated scoring machines that do the scoring for the bowler, but that should not preclude each bowler knowing how to score manually and knowing what constitutes a legal ball delivery. Therefore, the following information is a necessity for every bowler to know and to be able to perform.

The game or line of bowling consists of 10 frames. A bowler gets a maximum of two ball deliveries in each frame to knock all of the pins down. A perfect 300 game is scored by knocking all of the pins down with the first ball roll of each frame.

A typical scoresheet used in bowling is divided into the 10 frames. An accumulation score of each frame is kept, to come up with the final game score. In the top right corner of each frame is a pair of small boxes, one for each ball roll.

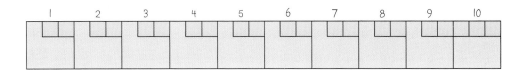

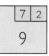

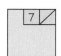

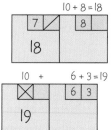

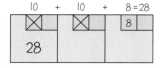

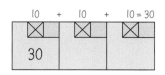

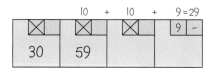

The pinfall on each ball delivery is entered in the little boxes. If a bowler knocks down 7 pins on the first delivery, a 7 is placed in the first box.

If on the second ball, the bowler knocks 2 of the remaining 3 pins down, a 2 is placed in the second little box and the total fall for both balls is recorded in the frame.

If the bowler knocks down all of the pins in a frame in *two* deliveries, a spare is the result and is recorded by placing a diagonal slash (/) in the second little box.

To score a spare, the bowler will receive the 10 pins knocked down in that frame plus the pinfall of the next single ball delivery.

If a bowler knocks down all the pins with the first ball, it is called a strike and is recorded in the first little box as an X. In case of a strike, the second ball is not needed because all of the pins are already knocked down. A bowler who is credited with a strike gets to score the 10 pins he or she knocked down with that ball plus a bonus of the pinfall on the next two deliveries. Therefore, if a strike is recorded, nothing is placed in that frame until that bowler's turn comes up again and he or she rolls the next two balls for the next frame or frames.

If the bowler records two strikes in a row, it is called a "double." To figure the pin count, follow the rule of 10 plus the next 2 balls. In this case, count the 10 pins knocked down by the strike ball, the ten on the first bonus ball, and the eight on the second bonus ball.

If a bowler rolls 3 strikes in a row, it is called a triple or a "turkey." Again, follow the rule of the 10 plus the pin count from the next two ball rolls, which will result in a total of 30.

Then, using the same formula, figure the score for a double and add to the previous frame score.

Now figure the score for the single strike left.

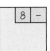

And finally, add the 9 pin count for the next frame.

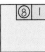

Self Evaluation QUESTIONS ?

1. Explain the basic formula for figuring
   a. spares
   b. strikes

2. Score the following:

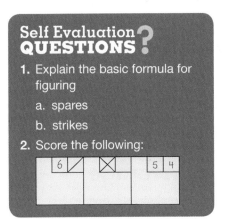

If a bowler fails to knock any pins down on a ball roll, a miss (-) is recorded in the respective corner square.

When the pins left following the first delivery constitute a split, a circle is drawn around the number of pins knocked down on that delivery. The pins knocked down on the second ball roll are still recorded in the little right hand box.

If a bowler fouls on the first delivery of a frame, an F is recorded in the first little box and no pinfall is counted. All of the pins are reset for the second ball delivery. Only the pins knocked down with the second ball are counted; in this case, 6 pins were knocked down.

If, after knocking down pins on the first ball of a frame, a foul is made, an F is recorded in the second little box and only the pinfall of the first ball delivery is counted in that frame.

The 10th frame is the final frame of the game. It is scored exactly as the previously scored frames unless a strike or spare occurs. When a spare occurs in the 10th frame, one bonus ball must be rolled to find out how much the spare scores. In this case, 10 (the pins knocked down in the spare) plus the 8 pins knocked down with the bonus ball. The 18-pin count is then added to the total in the 9th frame and placed in the 10th. **That is the end of the game.**

When a strike is recorded in the 10th frame, the bowler must roll two more balls to find out how much that strike scores. The score for the last strike (18) is added to the 9th frame

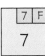

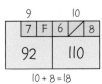

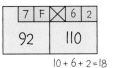

Self Evaluation QUESTIONS ?

1. Explain the basic formula for figuring the score for a strike in the 10th frame.

2. How is a split indicated on the score sheet?

3. Score the following 10th frame

10	TOTAL
124	124
136	260
103	363

score. The total score placed in the 10th frame is the score of the game, and the pinfall from the extra two ball rolls is not added on.

The total column at the end of each line is used to total accumulated game scores. This score constitutes the bowler's series score.

Here is an example of an individual game:

1	2	3	4	5	6	7	8	9	10
7 2	5 /	8 /	⊠	4 3	⊠	⊠	6 /	8 –	⊠ ⊠ 5
9	27	47	64	71	97	117	135	143	168

How to Calculate an Average

124
136
103
100
152
134
169
122
180
1220 ÷ 9 = 135 average

If the total series is divided by the number of games bowled, the bowler's average for the series is obtained (e.g., 363 ÷ 3 = 121). During a competitive season, a bowler keeps a running account of his or her current average. This is accomplished by keeping track of each game bowled and adding it to the cumulative total of games previously bowled. By continually totaling and dividing the total by the number of games bowled, the bowler will find his or her current average. Any extra pins left over (fractions) are dropped from the average.

Self Evaluation QUESTIONS ?

1. What is Kelly's average after bowling the following four games? 100, 162, 171, 203

2. What happens if there are pins left over when figuring an average?

Basic Rules of Bowling

The following is a summary of rules and regulations in the game of bowling as established by the United States Bowling Congress:

- In league play, a team shall start bowling on the lane for which it is scheduled. The team then alternates lanes with the paired lane for each succeeding frame. The second game is started on the paired lane.
- A ball is legally delivered when it leaves the bowler's possession and crosses the foul line into playing territory.
- During or after the delivery, if any part of a bowler touches beyond the foul line, it constitutes a foul. The following are other interpretations concerning fouls:

  1. Touching a wall, post, or other structure, unless local ground rules are established, also constitutes a foul.
  2. When any foreign object drops from a bowler (e.g., keys, cap, jewelry, pens, and so on) on or across the foul, the bowler should signal the scorer or opposing team before picking up the dropped article to avoid any possibility of being charged with a foul.
  3. If the bowler's hand or any other body part touches the lane beyond the foul line, a foul must be called. This is true even if the foul detecting device did not register the foul.
  4. If the bowler's foot (or any other part of the body) crosses the foul line on an adjacent lane, a foul must be recorded.
  5. A foul cannot be called when the ball rolls over the foul line during delivery.
  6. A foul is not committed when a bowler crosses the foul line but retains possession of the ball.

- If a bowler fouls on the first ball delivery of a frame, the pins knocked down do not count and all of the pins are reset for the second ball delivery. Only the pins knocked down on the second ball roll count. If a bowler does knock all 10 pins down with the second ball, it is recorded as a spare.
- If a bowler fouls on the second ball of a frame, only the pin count from the first ball roll is recorded.
- Pins knocked down by a ball that first falls into the channel do not count. If this occurs on the first roll of a frame, this pin(s) must be reset before the next ball delivery.
- Pins that are moved off to the side or bounce off the lane and back again, but remain standing, are considered as pins standing. If any standing pin is knocked down by the pinsetter, it must be placed into position before the next ball roll.
- All deadwood (pins knocked down) must be cleared from the lane before the next ball is delivered.
- Pins knocked over by a ball rebounding off the rear cushion do not count.
- In the case of a "dead ball," that ball shall not count and the pins shall be respotted for a rebowl situation. The following are situations where a "dead ball" is declared:

  1. There is interference with the ball before it reaches the pins.
  2. One or more pins are missing from the set-up.
  3. Bowling on the wrong lane or out of turn.
  4. When a player is interfered with before the delivery is completed, providing the bowler immediately calls attention to the fact.
  5. A pin is interfered with before the ball reaches it.

In a Nutshell

- A perfect game in bowling (all strikes) results in a 300 game.
- There are 10 frames in a line (or game) of bowling.
- You get two ball rolls each frame to knock down the 10 pins.
- If you knock down all 10 pins with the two ball rolls, it is called a spare and is worth the 10 pins you knocked down plus the pins knocked down on the next ball delivery in the next frame.
- If you knock all the pins down with just one ball delivery, it is called a strike and is worth the 10 pins you knocked down plus the total of the next two balls delivered in the next frame.
- The total score appearing in the 10th frame is the score for the game.
- An average is figured by taking the accumulative total of all games divided by the number of games completed.
- Adherence to the rules of bowling is a must for all bowling participants.

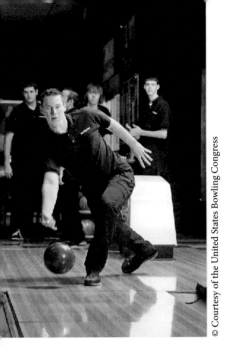

League Bowling

Some 7 million people a year bowl in some type of sanctioned league throughout the U.S. The following information is presented in this text to give a better understanding of the various elements associated with league bowling.

Types of Leagues

A league is usually defined as four or more competitive teams bowling a prearranged schedule. Each team is usually made up of three or four bowlers. One of the members of each team is designated as a team captain. Among the responsibilities of this captain are the team's conduct, accuracy of the league sheets for the team, handicapping of the team, collection of the money, and completion of the forms at the end of each day of competition.

There are two major kinds of leagues in bowling: the scratch league and the handicap league. The scratch league merely means that the actual scores rolled by the bowlers are the scores used in competition. There is no means of equalizing the scores of the bowlers by giving pins to the less-skilled bowler.

The handicap league "gives" pins to less-skilled bowlers to equalize their abilities, thus providing better, closer competition. Each league establishes its own handicap formula to be used throughout the season.

Handicapping

There are two main kinds of handicapping: the individual base handicap and the team base handicap. Each league will decide which of these styles of handicapping will be used, and what base and percentage to use.

The Base Score

The base from which a handicap is figured is usually established by looking at the league's top bowler(s). The base should usually be a little above the top bowler(s) in the league. For leagues with bowlers who average in the 180s and 190s, a 200 base is commonly established. This basically means that a 200 average bowler would be bowling scratch, no handicap. Any bowler under a 200 would get a percentage of the pin difference between his or her average and the handicap base. In a lesser skilled league where the top bowler(s) does not exceed the average of 170 or so, a 180 base may be selected.

The Selected Percentage

To merely subtract a bowler's average from the base score would not be quite fair. Therefore, a designated percentage of the difference between the bowler's average and the base score is identified. The most common percentages are probably 75 and 80 percent, but they may range from 60 to 100.

Figuring Individual Base Handicaps

Some leagues will require that the handicap be figured for each individual on the team. Suppose the league has selected a base score of 180 and an 80 percent handicap figure. The following procedure would be followed to find Sam's handicap per game when he has an average of 140.

		Individual Handicap
Example:	Sam	32
	Jane	40
	Tony	14
	Sue	10
	Jerry	12
		108 pins

		Average		
Example:	Sam	140	900	Team Base
	Jane	130	−765	Team Total Average
	Tony	162	135	
	Sue	168	× .80	
	Jerry	165	108.00	Pins
		765		

Subtract Sam's average from the base score.

Then take 80 percent of that number.

For each game Sam rolls, 32 pins will be added to his score.

```
  180
 −140
   40
 × .80
 32.00
```

To find a team's handicap for each game using this system, each team member's handicap is figured, as was Sam's, and added together.

This team would have a team handicap of 108 pins per game.

Team Base Handicapping

Sometimes it is more convenient to figure the total team handicap all in a single calculation rather than five separate calculations for each of the team members. This is accomplished by finding the team base by multiplying the 180 base score by the number of team members (180 × 5 = 900). This team base score, once found, will remain 900 throughout the season.

Now add all of the team members' averages together, subtract that total from the team base of 900, and take 80 percent of the difference.

Each week the handicap will differ from the week before because the individual averages will change.

Figuring Marks

In competitive bowling, a player or a team is interested in knowing the status of its score in relation to its opponents' as the game progresses. Instead of totaling each frame, an easy system has been worked out where marks are counted. A strike or a spare is usually

Self Evaluation QUESTIONS

1. If Jon is in a 200 base handicap league where they use 75 percent difference in figuring handicaps, what is his handicap per game if he has a 150 average one particular night?
2. How is a team handicap calculated?
3. What is a "scratch" league?

	1	2	3	4	5	6	7	8	9	10	
TEAM	9 - → 9	5 / → 25	6 2 → 33	⑦ 2 → 42	F 8 → 50	9 / → 70	X → 89	8 1 → 98	6 2 → 106	X 3 6 → 125	125
A	X → 19	8 1 → 28	6 - → 34	X → 62	X → 80	8 - → 88	8 1 → 97	5 2 → 104	X → 124	7 / 8 → 142	267
(MARKS)	1	2	–	3 + 1	5	6	7	–	8	10	
TEAM	6 2 → 8	9 - → 17	6 / → 35	8 - → 43	X → 62	4 5 → 71	8 / → 86	5 3 → 94	F 6 → 100	9 - → 109	109
B	6 3 → 9	2 / → 27	⑧ - → 35	X → 51	3 3 → 57	9 - → 66	4 / → 84	8 - → 92	X → 112	5 / 6 → 128	237
(MARKS)	1	2	3	4	–	6	–	7	8		

referred to as a mark, and each mark is worth a value of 10 pins. By counting the marks in each frame and keeping a running total, the bowler can tell approximately how many pins ahead or behind he or she is in that game. Example above:

By examining the marks in frame 2, Team A has one mark more than Team B, which is approximately 10 pins. In the 7th frame, Team A has 7 to Team B's six marks, a difference of one mark or approximately 10 pins. At that point Team A knows that they have about 10 pins more than Team B without looking at the scores. At the end of the game Team A has two marks more than Team B, so they will win by approximately 20 pins.

This system is more commonly used in league bowling because team progress is difficult to figure because of the five different scores.

After each complete frame, the scorer adds the total marks to that point of the total team.

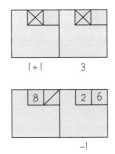

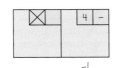

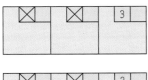

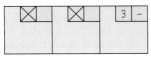

Mark Guidelines

- To receive a mark, it is necessary for a player to get a strike or a spare.
- To gain two marks in a frame, it is necessary for a player to get two strikes in a row.
- Four ways of losing marks are:

1. Following a spare, with the next ball the bowler knocks down fewer than 5 pins.
2. Following a strike, the bowler knocks down fewer than 5 pins in two attempts.
3. Following a double, the bowler rolls the next ball and knocks down fewer than 5 pins.
4. Following a double, the bowler knocks down fewer than 5 pins total on two ball deliveries. *Loss of two marks.*

Figuring Team Handicap Differences into Marks

At the start of the first game, each team finds its handicap. The team handicaps are then compared to determine the pin difference, if any.

Should one team have six or more pins greater handicap than the other, the difference is converted into marks (i.e., the difference is divided by 10). This number of marks is then recorded on the lower left edge of the scoresheet to indicate the advantage one team has at the start of the game.

Cumulative marks are then recorded for each game in each frame to allow the teams to see their competitive progress throughout the game. In this way, a team can tell how far ahead or behind they are at the end of any given frame.

In figuring marks from the handicap, if the figure comes out to a fraction, round it off to the closest number. This is the only time any numbers are rounded off. In all cases of figuring averages and/or handicaps, any extra pins or fractions are dropped.

Mark Chart for Various Game Scores

The following chart indicates how many marks (strikes and spares) are normally required to reach different scores. A maximum score of only 90 is possible without making a spare or strike. And it is impossible to bowl over 200 without having two strikes together.

To Score:	Marks Required:
91–103	1
104–113	2
114–123	3
124–133	4
134–143	5
144–153	6
154–163	7
164–173	8
174–183	9
184 & Over	10

Tardy Bowler

It is common courtesy for bowlers to be at the establishment ready to bowl at the designated time. However, there are circumstances that may prevent a person from arriving on time. If this does occur in league bowling, usually a bowler who arrives before the end of the third frame is allowed to catch up. If he/she arrives after the third frame has been completed, the team is obligated to make that person sit out for the remainder of that game and be given a "blind score."

Absent League Bowler

Each league establishes a "blind score" or "dummy" score in case a member of a team is absent. The most commonly used blind score is found by taking the absent bowler's current average minus 10, which is his or her game score. By using the aforementioned mark chart, the team may count marks according to the blind score to keep the mark count accurate.

Setting Up a League Schedule

In setting up a league schedule, the most important factor to consider is to make sure each team gets an equal chance. This is accomplished by making sure that the teams rotate lanes each session and that each team gets to roll against all other teams an equal number of times.

Lane assignments can be made for the entire league schedule the first day of the league. The following are single round robin schedules for leagues with 6, 8, 10, or 12 teams, respectively.

League Lane Assignments

6 Team Schedule Insert Lane Numbers			
DATE			
	Team Code Numbers		
1	1-2	3-4	5-6
2	3-5	2-6	1-4
3	1-6	2-3	4-5
4	4-2	1-5	6-3
5	6-4	1-3	5-2

League Lane Assignments   **8 Team Schedule**

Insert Lane Numbers

DATE				
	Team Code Numbers			
1	1-2	3-4	5-6	7-8
2	6-8	5-7	2-4	1-3
3	5-4	1-8	7-3	2-6
4	3-6	7-2	1-5	8-4
5	7-1	4-6	3-8	5-2
6	2-3	8-5	4-1	6-7
7	4-7	6-1	8-2	3-5

League Lane Assignments   **10 Team Schedule**

Insert Lane Numbers

DATE					
	Team Code Numbers				
1	1-2	3-4	5-6	7-8	9-10
2	7-3	1-6	2-9	5-10	8-4
3	4-5	9-8	10-1	3-2	6-7
4	9-1	5-3	4-7	8-6	10-2
5	10-7	6-2	8-3	4-1	5-9
6	5-8	10-4	7-2	6-9	1-3
7	6-4	7-9	1-5	10-3	2-8
8	3-9	8-1	6-10	2-4	7-5
9	8-10	2-5	9-4	1-7	3-6

League Lane Assignments   **12 Team Schedule**

Insert Lane Numbers

DATE						
	Team Code Numbers					
1	1-2	3-4	5-6	7-8	9-10	11-12
2	4-5	6-2	12-3	9-11	1-7	10-8
3	9-3	1-10	11-4	5-12	8-2	6-7
4	7-12	5-8	9-2	10-4	11-6	1-3
5	11-8	9-7	1-5	6-3	10-12	2-4
6	10-6	11-1	3-8	12-2	7-4	9-5
7	5-7	4-12	2-10	1-9	6-8	3-11
8	12-9	10-5	7-11	4-6	2-3	8-1
9	6-1	2-11	8-12	3-5	4-9	7-10
10	3-10	8-9	4-1	2-7	5-11	12-6
11	8-4	7-3	6-9	11-10	12-1	5-2

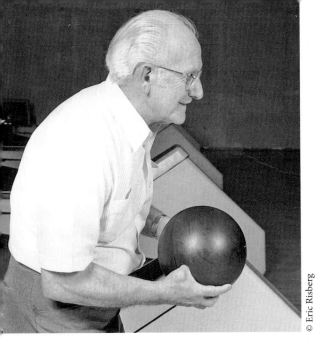
© Eric Risberg

Bowling for Those with Special Needs

In recent years, enormous strides have taken place in our society to provide recreational services for our special populations. Two special-needs groups will be addressed in this chapter of the bowling text—the senior bowler and those with disabilities.

The Senior Bowler

Due to better health care and active lifestyles, the fastest growing group of those with special needs in the United States is the senior citizen. Our seniors are now a very physically active group. Recreational services for this population have grown dramatically in the past decade, providing them with a variety of activities to meet their needs, interests, and abilities (Figure 10.1). One of the best lifetime activities that has ease of modification, if needed, is the sport of bowling. A variety of bowling activities and programs are readily available for the senior. The following are some tips for the senior bowler.

Tips for the Senior Bowler

Often a senior bowler has a need to work around physical impairments, injuries, phobias, and misconceptions.

Sticking to the fundamentals of an activity is not always possible, so adjustments need to be made, taking into account what the bowler physically can or cannot do. Emphasis should be placed on the bowler's strengths (e.g., improving the follow-through when the knee bend cannot be achieved). Also, consideration must be given to the number of games that a senior can bowl at one time (three may be too many). Some special tips for the senior bowler include:

1. Select a bowling ball that is not too heavy. It is better to use a ball that is too light than one that is too heavy, to keep from tiring too fast. Even if a bowler has bowled for many years, it is important to decrease the weight of the ball to help maintain a consistent ball speed. Often seniors have difficulty acknowledging that they need to decrease ball weight (Figure 10.2).

2. It is strongly advised that seniors use a conventional grip and avoid a fingertip grip. There is less physical strain on the hand using a conventional grip (Figure 10.3).

3. For physical impairments involving the hand, extra holes should be drilled in the ball

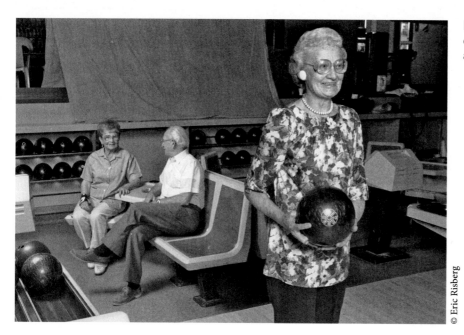

FIGURE 10.1 Seniors can find physical activity and enjoyment in bowling.

© Eric Risberg

on the ball, but would gain better control of the ball at the release point.

4. For a newcomer to bowling, it would be best to concentrate on a one- or two-step approach. Often seniors have difficulty in coordinating the armswing with the footwork. By taking fewer steps, effort can be placed on the pendulum swing and release, eliminating thoughts about footwork.

A zero-step approach can be employed if there are serious leg or back problems. However, in all of these adjustments, a lack of speed could be a potential shortcoming (Figure 10.4).

for gripping purposes. This does not create an illegal bowling ball, as the rules of ABC allow for as many holes to be drilled in the ball as required for gripping purposes. The bowler may sacrifice lift

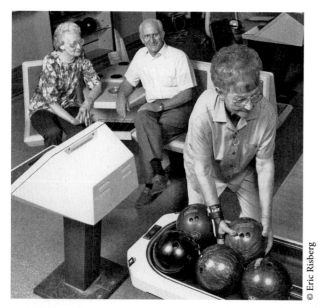

FIGURE 10.2 Remember to pick the ball up from the return with both hands and face the pins.

© Eric Risberg

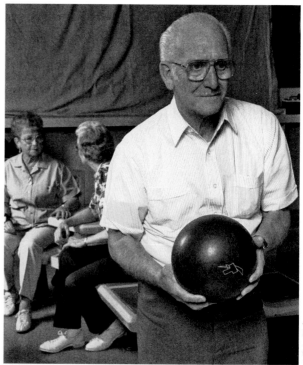

FIGURE 10.3 A senior should use a fingertip grip only if his or her skill and physical capabilities allow.

© Eric Risberg

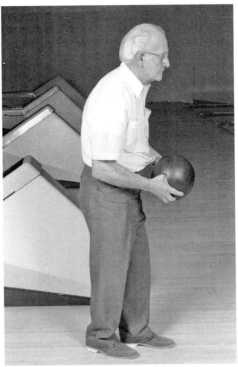

FIGURE 10.4   Taking fewer steps and starting the approach closer to the foul line can help coordination.

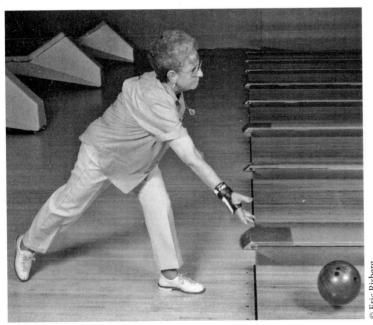

FIGURE 10.5   Leaning forward more can help a senior who has difficulty with knee bend.

5. If the swing and release can be mastered, then a four-step approach could be tried.

6. A common problem is an inability to bend the knees at the foul line. If this is the case, the bowler should lean forward more at the release point to avoid lofting the ball. Without knee bend, there is greater tendency to turn the shoulders and hips away from the target and to pull the ball across the body at release. To counteract this tendency, the bowler needs to focus on a straight armswing and follow-through down the lane to the target (Figure 10.5).

7. A key point for seniors is to learn how to adjust to lane conditions. Most tend to roll the ball very slowly, which allows the lane to have more time to take the ball away from

its intended path. To compensate for this lack of speed, the bowler must be especially conscious of turning the body to face the target or the intended objective.

8. Emphasis must be placed on the follow-through. The follow-through must always go in the same direction and to the same level (Figure 10.6).

9. In terms of selecting a target, a senior bowler can still use the dots and arrows that other bowlers use along with the strike and spare adjustment systems. However, it is not an error to be a pin bowler. If this method is used, the bowling shoulder needs to be aligned and turned in the direction of the objective (Figure 10.7).

10. For those with vision problems, using the dots which are 7 feet forward of the foul line could be helpful for a closer aiming point. However, the closer one's target, the greater the tendency to bend too much from the waist and have a low follow-through.

11. For a senior who is just beginning to bowl, it is best to deliver the ball so that the thumb points toward the pins (Figure 10.8). The attempt here is to roll a straight ball and to avoid too much roll or hook to the left or to the right. Because of the lack of speed, the bowler needs to concentrate on keeping the swing and ball "on line." A hook ball is not a necessity.

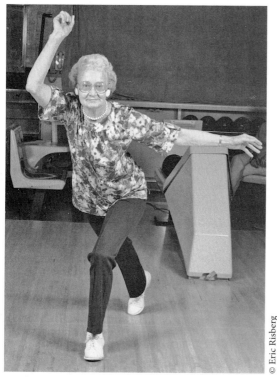

© Eric Risberg

FIGURE 10.6   A consistent follow-through is a key to accuracy.

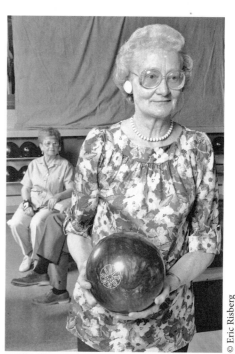

© Eric Risberg

FIGURE 10.7   Whichever target is chosen, keep the eyes focused on that target throughout the approach and delivery.

12. To increase consistency, upon the release of the ball, the senior should be conscious of trying to keep the body as still as possible. The only thing that should move is the arm traveling into its natural follow-through. This tip assists in maintaining balance and concentrating on the target.

13. Often with seniors, the conventional "rules" concerning fundamentals do not apply. The rules need to be bent to overcome a lack of stamina and strength. There is often a need for individual adjustments and "styles" to counteract physical difficulties (Figures 10.9 and 10.10). There are a variety of disabling conditions, and it would be impossible to cover all of these conditions and

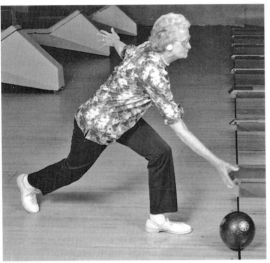

FIGURE 10.8   Delivering the ball with the thumb pointing toward the pins helps the ball stay on course.

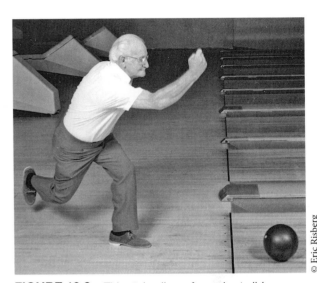

FIGURE 10.9   This style allows for a short slide.

FIGURE 10.10   This senior finds less strain on his arms by holding the ball centered in the stance.

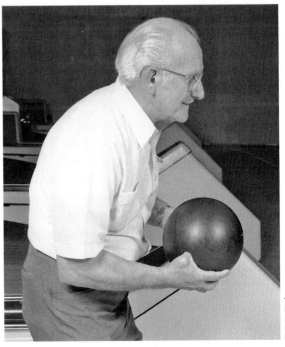

the bowling adaptations that would have to be made to treat each unique situation. This would be another book in itself. So it is the authors' intent in this section to give a general overview of guidelines that may benefit those with disabilities and those assisting them.

Bowling for Those with Disabilities

In recent years, our society has made a concerted effort to bring people with disabilities into the mainstream and into recreational activities. Many of those with disabilities will be able to enjoy the game of bowling without any modifications. Others may need assistance with equipment, or modifications must be made and provided. With the movement of inclusion, many bowling establishments have encouraged those with disabilities to enjoy the challenge of bowling by providing an environment with adaptive devices and equipment to meet the needs of these special bowlers.

Guidelines for Those with Disabilities

1. Select a bowling ball that is not too heavy.
2. A bowling ball with a conventional grip is advised.
3. A one- or two-step approach may be acceptable in many cases.
4. A straight ball release is encouraged for many, but a hook ball is still desirable in many instances.
5. Emphasis is on the delivery and follow-through. Emphasize leaning forward and placing the ball on the lane and following through completely toward the target.
6. Pin bowling may take the place of spot or target bowling. However, if possible, incorporate spot bowling into the bowling fundamentals.
7. To have a measure of success, adaptive devices and equipment are occasionally available at the bowling establishment.
8. Make sure that only one player at a time is on the approach. When not bowling, stay in the settee area.
9. Keep the hands away from the ball return, especially where the ball pops up.

Guidelines for Instructing Those with Disabilities

1. It would be highly advisable to have one-to-one assistance while keeping the groups small.
2. Determine the abilities of each individual and identify the needs and realistic goals for each.
3. In reaching these goals, develop a simple plan of attack and then keep things simple.
4. Keeping things fun is important as ample practice is given to each segment of the skill.
5. Modifications of the game may occur, but most want to play the game/activity the way everyone else does.
6. Each will have a level where he or she is functioning. Many will have to start at the lowest skill level, whereas many may be at a higher level.
7. Each needs to have maximum activity with a minimum of passive time.
8. Each needs praise and lots of celebration!

Examples of adaptive bowling equipment include handle-grip bowling balls where the handles automatically retract into the ball upon delivery; bowling rails to guide the visually impaired; adjustable ball release bowling ramps where the ball is placed atop and then pushed down in the direction of the pins; and channel bumpers to prevent balls from entering the channel while traveling toward the pins.

For those who do not need adaptive equipment and would like to enjoy the game of bowling on their own but may need slight modifications, we suggest following the previous guidelines written for the senior bowler. By choosing the suggestions that pertain directly to your needs, you will be able to enjoy an afternoon of bowling at your favorite establishment. (For additional information on teaching bowling to the disabled, see the Instructor's Manual.)

Bowling and Pregnancy

There is no reason why a pregnancy should interrupt the enjoyment of the game of bowling. However, it is strongly advised that pregnant bowlers get a physician's release before engaging in the sport of bowling. Most bowlers will very likely be granted this permission and will be able to continue bowling throughout the pregnancy unless there are complications associated with the pregnancy. It is possible during the last month or two that fatigue and the tired back syndrome may limit the bowling of some.

For a pregnant woman engaging in the activity of bowling, there will be a few physical changes that may affect bowling. First of all, the vertical balance line may be slightly skewed, finding the bowler more upright or leaning slightly backward in the approach and delivery. To counter this, it is important to accentuate the arm going farther out toward the target arrow so the release of the ball is farther out on the lane than what seems natural.

Secondly, the legs will have a tendency to tire more easily. Those taking the game seriously might need to do additional leg strengthening exercises. If the legs do get tired during the games, the knee bend at the release point will be less. Therefore, it is really necessary that the arm again reach out as far as possible to the target to help counter the more upright position of the bowler at the time of the delivery.

Probably the most important element that can be stressed for a pregnant bowler is to guard against additional back pain while participating in bowling. Several suggestions are in order to assist in this endeavor: (1) Avoid carrying bowling equipment long distances. It is advised that a bowler get a bag that has wheels. (2) Always pick up a bowling ball, whether from the bag, racks, or ball return, with hands around the ball and knees bent. Use the straightening of the knees to lift the ball and not the back. (3) When delivering the ball, bend those knees! This will get the body lower on the delivery and will assist in taking the strain of the weight of the ball away from the back.

There is also a possibility that the swing may be affected due to the pregnancy. It is advised that, in the stance, the ball be held slightly off to the side (rather than at the center of the body) to emphasize that the pushaway be in line with the ensuing pendular swing. This should keep everything in a straight line going toward the target arrow.

There is no reason that a pregnant woman cannot enjoy the sport of bowling. Many women will find that they actually will improve their averages during this time, possibly due to a slower, more cautious foot speed on the approach and greater concentration on the balance at the line. Others will find it a bit more challenging. Regardless, the excitement and social aspects of bowling will remain. So after your physician's clearance, go for it!

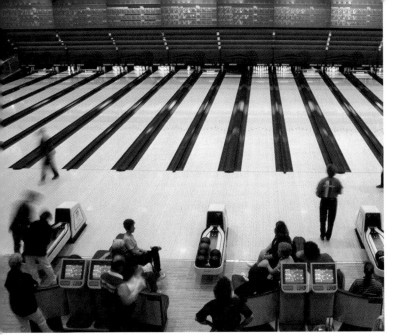

© Mark E. Gibson/Documentary/CORBIS

11

The Modern Bowling Environment

The entire world has been affected by the rapid changes in technology and the development of new materials. Bowling is no exception. In the last twenty years, many changes have taken place in the game of bowling. These changes range from synthetic pins and lanes to new ball surfaces that are capable of being adjusted to the particular lane conditions and oiling systems. The traditional wooden lanes and familiar balls are rapidly disappearing. With the modern changes, bowlers must be prepared (both physically and mentally) to face a bowling environment that may have greater variations and pose new challenges. In this chapter, we hope to give you a glimpse of the modern bowling environment and many of the changes that may be occurring as we enter the twenty-first century.

Lanes and Lane Conditions

Whether the lanes are wooden or synthetic, one of the most crucial variables a bowler must deal with is the variation in lane conditions from lane to lane, day to day, and from establishment to establishment. Lane conditions will change even from the start of a bowling session to the end. The capability of a bowler to make adjustments to correspond with the lane condition at the time will determine the difference between a good performance and a bad performance. Whereas we have previously indicated several adjustment systems that can be used to adjust to the varying lane conditions, a little information on lane conditions may prove helpful at this time.

As you may guess, the bowling lane surface is subject to a considerable amount of daily play and "wear and tear." To minimize the wear and tear, to equalize lane conditions, and to prevent damage to the surface of the lanes, bowling establishments carefully maintain the lane surfaces. Most establishments care for their lanes on a daily basis. A very thin coat of oil-based "dressing" is applied to the lane surface, which helps protect the lane from the balls traveling on it, somewhat as a motor oil protects a car's engine. Oiling machines are now very high tech. They operate on the same principle as an ink-jet printer in that the volume and pattern of oil placed on each single board is predetermined through a computer-type program. In modern bowling establishments, there are two commonly used oiling patterns, commonly known as the Christmas Tree Pattern and the Top Hat Pattern. Each of these patterns will have a different effect on a bowling ball traveling toward the pins. It is advised that bowlers check with their usual bowling establishment, which can provide more in-depth knowledge as to which pattern they are using and how it is applied. This knowledge can then be used in adjusting one's point of origin or point of aim.

Fast Lanes

With the different application systems, amounts of oil, and patterns of lane oiling, we find lanes that will vary a great deal, which will affect the ball roll. The greater the quantity of oil applied to the lane, the more the ball tends to skid on its path to the pins. Because of the skid of the ball, it will not "grab" or hook soon enough for the proper angle of entry into the pins. This is usually called a **"fast lane"** or **"oily lane."** Adjustments must take place to enable the ball to break sooner, which is usually done by moving the point of origin in your stance farther right (right handers) or farther left (left handers) (see Chapter 6—3-1-2 Strike Adjustment System).

Slow or Hooking Lanes

The lane with less oil, called a **"slow"** or **hooking lane**, allows the ball to hook more. It actually skids less, which allows the ball to begin its roll sooner on the lane. The angle of entry into the pocket generally needs to be decreased by the bowler on this type of lane, so the adjustment for a right-handed bowler would be to generally move his or her point of origin slightly to the left, whereas a left-handed bowler would move his or her point of origin slightly to the right (see Chapter 6—3-1-2 Strike Adjustment System). Another adjustment could be to select a "stronger" ball.

Today's Lanes

According to the United States Bowling Congress, today's lanes must have a minimum of three "units" of dressing applied across the lane for any distance that the lane is dressed. The general effect of this rule should be that the bowler might feel that the lane is oilier and that the ball does not hook as much. It is the bowler's ability to adapt to changing lane conditions that will determine the eventual game score. This process is called "reading the lane" to determine just what adjustments in the target or point of origin may be necessary. Remember that the approach, armswing, and delivery should remain consistent no matter what the lane conditions are like. The correct adjustment to the appropriate strike line will mean the difference between a successful performance or a frustrating one.

Newest Trends in Lanes Found in 21st Century Bowling Establishments

- Even though about 40 percent of the bowling lanes are still made of wood, all recently installed lanes are synthetic and have a laminate surface.
- The new synthetic Brunswick lanes have an additional marking on the lane to assist the "modern" player. Four dark boards (each about 3 feet long) have been added about two-thirds of the way down the lane (or about 40 feet). Two are placed on the right and the other two on the left. The purpose of these additional targets is to assist the modern player in judging the **"break point"** (the point where the ball stops sliding and starts its move to the pins—usually the

FIGURE 11.1   Break point in a ball roll.

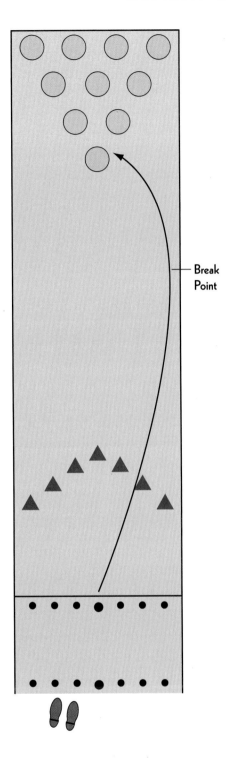

Break Point

up into the gutters, preventing gutter balls and allowing everyone to enjoy knocking down pins.

- **"Cosmic Bowling,"** where lanes actually glow due to an ultraviolet additive to the lane dressing, is popular now in recreational bowling.

- **USBC** has developed a new program called "Sport Bowling," where lane conditions and equipment are more controlled, with the purpose of placing more emphasis on a bowler's advanced skill. This is an attempt to decrease the assistance given bowlers from the lane condition and high tech bowling balls. In the United States, leagues are being formed that will bowl on Sport Bowling lane conditions. The PBA (Professional Bowler's Association) holds its tournaments on these lane conditions, along with all major international amateur organizations and championships.

- Under Sport Bowling conditions, shot-making is at a premium and a bowler is unable to get away with inconsistencies. Absolute command of one's game is needed. This move is meant to try to bring credibility and shot-making (different from accuracy) back to bowling.

- On a Sport Bowling lane, the lane conditions can vary a great deal due to the quantity and length of dressing down the lane. However, there may be no more than a 2:1 ratio of dressing anywhere on the lane side-to-side.

- A recreational bowler playing on Sport Bowling conditions can expect a 20-25 pin drop in his or her average. If a "sport bowler" has established an average on sport bowling lanes, the USBC has created a chart (Figure 11.2) for this bowler to use to determine his or her equivalent

widest point in the ball path) (Figure 11.1). These extra boards are used for targeting—to determine when and where the ball hooks.

- **"Bumpers,"** which are fillers in the channels (gutters) used by very young bowlers and those with special needs, are now built into the lanes. The bumpers rotate

adjusted average for recreational bowling. For example, if one who bowls in a Sport Bowling league has an average of 170, this average will be adjusted to 188 in a recreational league. A bowler cannot have an average adjusted downward (from recreational to sport); only upward (from sport to recreational).

Approaches

Today's synthetic lanes may find bowlers sensing that the approaches feel different. The approaches may feel more slippery than normal, or depending upon climate and humidity, they may feel stickier. Many of today's bowlers are electing to purchase an elite shoe that has removable/changeable

FIGURE 11.2   Sport league average adjustment to standard average chart.

SPORT LEAGUE AVERAGE	ADJUSTED AVERAGE	SPORT LEAGUE AVERAGE	ADJUSTED AVERAGE	SPORT LEAGUE AVERAGE	ADJUSTED AVERAGE
0-129	Same				
130	137	160	175	190	207
131	138	161	176	191	208
132	140	162	176	192	209
133	141	163	177	193	210
134	142	164	179	194	211
135	144	165	180	195	212
136	145	166	182	196	212
137	146	167	184	197	213
138	148	168	186	198	214
139	150	169	187	199	215
140	154	170	188	200	216
141	158	171	189	201	217
142	159	172	190	202	218
143	160	173	192	203	218
144	161	174	194	204	219
145	162	175	195	205	220
146	163	176	196	206	220
147	164	177	197	207	221
148	165	178	198	208	222
149	166	179	199	209	224
150	166	180	200	210	225
151	167	181	201	211	225
152	168	182	201	212	226
153	169	183	202	213	227
154	169	184	203	214	229
155	170	185	204	215	230
156	171	186	205	216	230
157	173	187	205	217	231
158	174	188	206	218	232
159	175	189	207	219 and up	SL Ave+15

soles and heels which can be used as a method of adjusting to approach conditions. However, the average bowler should be prepared to make his or her own adjustments with his or her shoes in order to compensate. The needed supplies to do this are listed at the end of this chapter.

Bowling Balls

Bowling balls have probably gone through the greatest changes in the last 20 years. Everyone is seeking that perfect ball to roll for that changing lane condition. This has resulted in new ball designs and ball covers every couple of years or months. The old rubber and plastic balls have been replaced by urethane and reactive resin balls. The urethane ball is more porous, grabs the lane more, and creates greater hook and hitting power. The reactive resin ball has a "sticky" feel to it and tends to have a greater reaction to the oilier and the drier parts of the lane. The newest ball on the market at the time of this printing is the resin with additive ball. This ball came on the market in 1998. It has a resin surface with very hard particles of material added to it. These balls tend to have a very smooth reaction (action is similar to all-season radial tires) and can be polished or sanded for the desired amount of hook (Figure 11.3).

The following is a summary of the four major types of bowling balls currently sought by bowlers:

1. Polyester (plastic)—This ball came on the market in the early 1960s. It is an attractive ball that today comes in many "collector novelty editions" such as Mickey Mouse, sport ball look-alikes (soccer, basketball, baseball), and clear balls with design inserts (flowers, logos, and so on). They range in price from $40 to $140.

2. Urethane—This type of ball came on the market in 1981. It is popular because the desired hook can be altered simply by sanding or polishing the surface. It ranges in price from $80 to $150.

3. Resin—This type of ball came on the market in 1991. The surface of the ball has a "sticky" feel and tends to have a greater reaction to the oilier and the drier parts of the lane. The surface of this ball can also be sanded or polished to the desired ball roll. They range in price from $80 to $280.

4. Resin with Additive—This ball came on the market in 1998. It has the resin surface with very hard particles of material added to it. These balls have a very smooth reaction and can also be polished or sanded for the desired hook. They range in price from $120 to $280.

Note: Bowling establishments may still use the old rubber balls as "house" balls.

The newer balls have resulted in bowlers readily increasing their averages by about 10 pins. The reason for

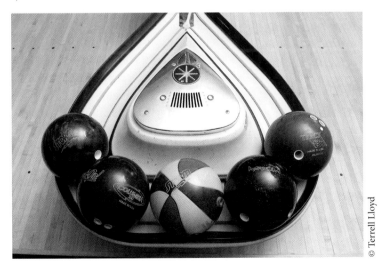

© Terrell Lloyd

FIGURE 11.3   Bowling balls are made of various materials; their surface can be dull or shiny.

this phenomenon is twofold: the reactive resin cover, and the density and shapes of the core of the ball. There are more manufacturers of bowling equipment today than ever before, and each is trying to improve and perfect ball cores. The cores come in ever-increasingly odd shapes. Two of them are illustrated: the light bulb-like shapes and the mushroom shapes (Figure 11.4). They may be symmetrical or asymmetrical. These cores, depending upon the design, affect the way the ball will react on the lane and against the pins.

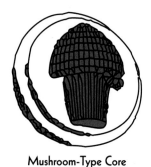

FIGURE 11.4 Ball cores come in different shapes.

Light Bulb-Type Core

Mushroom-Type Core

Ball Drilling

The professional who drills the ball must have specialized knowledge in the dynamics of each particular bowler's needs and the bowling ball itself. Professional expertise on the part of the ball driller is an absolute necessity. A bowling ball is no longer a simple round mass impacting 10 bowling pins. It has become a dynamic force that overpowers the pins. A ball's deflection has been greatly decreased. The older method of drilling in terms of the old idea of "weights" is no longer influential. In the ball weight method, the ball could only be drilled to create a maximum of a 4–6 inch difference in hook/roll pattern. However, the owner of a modern-day resin with additive ball can change the surface of the ball by sanding or polishing it to the point that the ball can change the hook/roll pattern by feet, not just inches. Therefore, this sanding or polishing of the reactive resin ball with different core structures has taken the place of "weights" or bowling ball "imbalances."

Automatic Scorers

Not every bowling center has automatic scoring devices, but you can readily recognize that a center has the automatic device when there are no lighted overhead projectors. Instead, you will see a television-type screen where the score is projected over the approach area (Figure 11.5).

Even with a machine that keeps score for the bowler, it is important to learn how to keep score, as that knowledge might be crucial in the outcome of a game (e.g., knowing what score a bowler needs to win). The major manufacturers have different types of automatic scoring systems (Figure 11.6). Upon entering the bowling center, the personnel at the control desk can provide you with

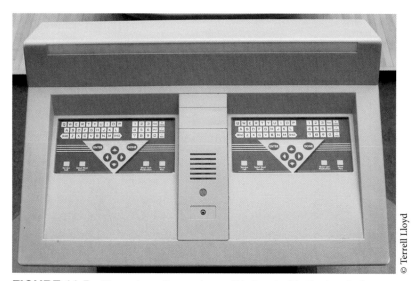

© Terrell Lloyd

FIGURE 11.5 The automatic scoring unit is located in the bowler's settee area.

the simple instructions required to make the scorer start. Most automatic scorers can be easily used by following the instructions printed or shown on the screen or the console. Corrections, adding of handicaps, or changes of information can be made manually by the bowler. Assistance can always be obtained from the personnel at the control desk.

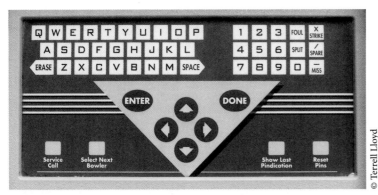

FIGURE 11.6 The bowler enters all necessary information into the machine and can also make scoring corrections.

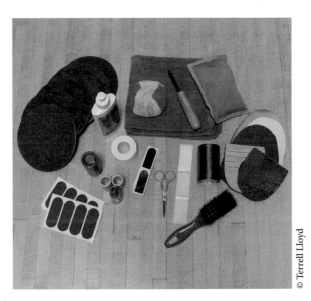

FIGURE 11.7 Some examples of a bowler's necessities.

Common Miscellaneous Bowling Supplies

To be prepared for the great variety of conditions and situations confronting the modern player, a bowler should have some supplies and aids available to him or her. The following supplies should be kept in a player's bowling bag and be available at a moment's notice (Figure 11.7).

For the bowling shoes:

Soapstone—can be applied to the bottom of the bowling shoe and help a bowler to have a smooth slide. Pencil lead or cigarette ashes can eliminate sticking in the same fashion. *Wire brush or coarse sandpaper*—to be used to rough up the soles for traction.

Note: Never use any powder on the bottoms of shoes or on the approaches.

Interchangeable soles—For the sliding shoe to easily adjust to different approach surfaces.

For the hand:

Cotton—for use with skin-patch. *Skin-patch*—a liquid to cover blisters, cuts, or tender spots on fingers.

Hand conditioner—to help the hand stay dry and get the same feel of the ball. This can come in a bag or jar, and can be a liquid or a powder.

Towel—to wipe the hand and/or the ball.

Wrist support—to support a weak wrist or lend extra support.

Lip balm or baby powder—for use on the thumb in extreme cases of swelling and a very fast thumb release. *Stretchable cloth thumb patch*—Protects thumb and fingers from abrasion; covers and protects injured areas. Also known as tape or a wrap.

For the ball:

Plastic tape—3/4" or 1" for use in adjusting the size of the thumb or finger holes as necessary. The tape can be cut to any length necessary and placed along the backside of the holes to make them more snug. The tape can be readily peeled away to make the hole larger.

Scissors—to cut the tape to needed lengths.

Emery board—to file down excessive build-up of calluses. *Fast drying glue*—for use on inserts or grips used in thumb or finger holes.

Round file or bevel knife—to repair edges of holes or enlarge them on the spot.

Alcohol—to clean thumb and finger holes from any kind of built-up residue and to clean the outside of the ball from a buildup of dirt or oil. The outside of the ball can only be cleaned prior to or after competition (not during).

Reactive resin ball cleaner—special liquid cleaner for reactive balls which tend to pick up dirt and oil due to their surface "tackiness" (available in pro shops).

Avalon pads™—Sanding pads used to alter the surface of a bowling ball; come in sets of grits ranging from 180 to 4000.

Finger Grips—Soft insert in finger holes used in most-fingertip grip bowling balls; can be replaced with different sizes or shapes (Round vs. Oval vs. Lip).

Molded thumb slug—A "premade" molded insert which has been created to the identical shape of a bowler's favorite thumb hole. Assists in making all bowling balls feel identical.

Interchangeable Thumb Insert—A slug drilled to a bowler's thumb shape preference which is interchangeable from one ball to another using a screw system. Assist in making all bowling equipment have the identical "Feel." Having these supplies readily on hand can help a bowler overcome distressful situations and continue bowling without a severe loss of pinfall. Without them, bowlers could find themselves in a situation where they might as well "call it a day."

The modern bowling environment in the twenty-first century does indeed require more than a ball, shoes, and a bowling lane. Knowledge and versatility are needed along with the ability to adapt to the ever-changing environments in which we find ourselves.

Electronic Bowling

Modern technologies have made many changes in how we now live our lives. Everyday a "new" product is being launched that is deemed "the best" and will change the world forever! Bowling has not escaped these changes, whether it is the bowling ball, the lane makeup and materials, the oiling systems, the handicap systems, or the automations in scoring. And now, the advent of electronic games has flooded the market and we find the inclusion of bowling in many of the game venues, and especially, in the television Wii game pack.

Are there any "carry-over" knowledge, concepts, and physical skills that can be learned through participation in these electronic games that can be transferred to the regular game of bowling? Absolutely. This will be examined in this segment of the book, but the instructional ideas and exercises will be found in the Instructor's Manual that accompanies the text.

Terminology and Knowledge Transfer

In these electronic bowling games, the knowledge and terminologies that players can learn through repetition and cognitive recognitions are (1) pin setup, (2) pin numbering, (3) pin action, (4) lane and approach markings and their relationship to one another, (5) spot bowling and the angles needed for spare conversions,

(6) scoring concepts, (7) strikes and spare terminology and concepts, (8) key pins for picking up spares, and (9) different hand positions for different ball rolls. The Wii also provides an avenue to competitive bowling whether it is against oneself or two or three others. Team bowling is also an option that leads right into league bowling. The limitations of electronic bowling in the learning of terminology and knowledge include the knowledge sets of proper etiquette, identification of key pins in spare leaves, and bowling terminology.

Physical Skill Transfer

Many of the skills that are all a part of bowling can be also practiced and learned while participating in electronic bowling. Participants can experiment with hand positions on ball releases and ball rolls. The last two steps, and definitely the last step, of the approach can be mastered with proper practice. That includes the balance lines, knee flexion, hip and shoulder action, the balance action of the non-bowling arm and back leg upon delivery and follow-though, and the release point and action of the hand, thumb, and arm. Speed control and proper spare and strike adjustment angles can be identified and practiced.

Please note: If the game of bowling is to be learned properly, it is paramount that the bowler take a class or have proper bowling instruction from a professional before engaging in electronic bowling for true bowling transfer. In this manner, the bowler will know precisely what techniques and knowledge he/she needs to concentrate on while practicing properly on a television game set. This precise practice will most definitely transfer to the regular game of bowling.

If a bowler is fortunate enough to have access to an electronic bowling game (especially on a large screen television), it can also be a cost-saving way of practicing. Along with all of the above benefits, it will have a built-in system that rewards good scores in various ways.

Bowling for All

Probably one of the greatest benefits of the electronic bowling games is the fact that all ages, all abilities, and all disabilities (including those in a wheelchair) can now enjoy the game of bowling from home or community center. It should be also noted that many senior-living communities are now sponsoring Wii bowling leagues. Minor adjustments can be made so everyone can learn, enjoy, and compete in the wonderful sport of bowling.

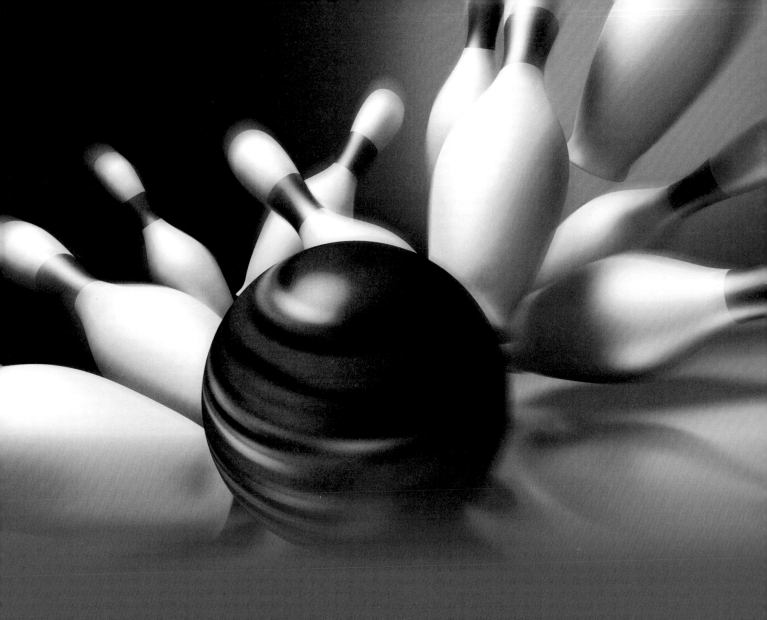

Advanced
BOWLING

PART**TWO**

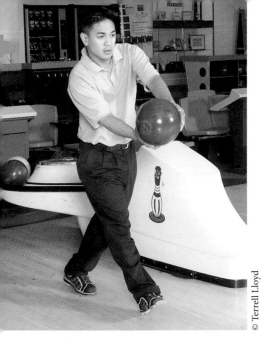

© Terrell Lloyd

12

Alternatives to the 4-Step Approach

For the purpose of establishing a common denominator in identifying an advanced bowler, we are making the assumption that advanced bowlers have a consistent and recognizable style and can carry an average over 140. Their experience gives them considerable background and knowledge.

Many times advanced bowlers hit a plateau and seem to be unable to raise their average. Because these bowlers have considerable experience in the game of bowling, and more than likely do many things well, they cannot erase their previous knowledge and start from scratch. Therefore, the next section of this text is devoted to improvements for advanced bowlers that should not destroy their existing game.

Suggested improvements, for the most part, will be minor; however, a few may be major. It should be noted that sometimes an old habit needs to be broken to make room for a better one. In such a case, the change might feel awkward and uncomfortable at first. Therefore, we urge the bowler to exercise patience and give suggested improvements a chance to work. Only then can the changes be reflected in improved scores.

After reaching a higher skill level, many bowlers start deviating from the norm and using techniques that seem to work best for them. They may vary the footwork patterns as well as their hand positions. We intend to provide a thorough understanding of these variations and suggest ideas for bettering what has been established or suggest the easiest method of change.

Footwork Variations

The **4-step approach** is the most common of all footwork patterns, mainly because it involves a natural rhythm where there is an arm motion for each foot motion. With this basic coordination, it is an easy and efficient approach to teach and to learn.

The first step of the 4-step approach is taken with the right foot for right handers and the left foot for left handers. Many bowlers have formed the habit of moving their arm and leg in opposition to one another and find it natural to step with the left foot. If this is the case, the bowler would develop a 3-, 5-, or 7-step approach.

Also, many bowlers feel the 4-step approach results in a choppy, robot-like movement, especially if they have learned it to a cadence of "one, two, three, and slide" instead of the "shuffle-shuffle-shuffle-slide" approach.

5-Step Approach

For many advanced bowlers, a **5-step approach** is fairly common. This 5-step approach allows for a more natural start because the right-handed bowler will step with the left foot (left-handed bowler with the right foot) using the principle of opposition where the legs and arms move in opposition to one another. The 5-step approach may also allow more time and distance in which to generate momentum on the ball. It gives the ball more time to move through the pendular swing.

The major disadvantage to this 5-step approach is the fact that there is not always a correlation between what the arms and feet are doing, making it more difficult to teach and learn. A bowler may also feel he or she must "rush to the foul line" to coordinate the ball and the feet at delivery.

Right-Handed Bowler and the 5-Step Approach

Actually the 5-step approach is similar to the 4-step approach, with the exception that the right-handed bowler's weight is on the right foot in the stance, but probably a little higher to allow for a little longer arc to take up the extra time of the extra step.

The ball is still pushed out and down in the pushaway after the left foot moves to counteract the weight of the ball. In other words, the bowler takes a small step with the left foot, then moves the ball in the second step. In contrast to the 4-step approach where the ball starts back on the *second* step, in the 5-step approach the ball is just starting into the backswing near the *third* step. With the additional length of the swing arc, the small extra step in the beginning should prevent any problems (Figures 12.1 and 12.2).

Left-Handed Bowler and the 5-Step Approach

Actually, the 5-step approach is similar to the 4-step approach, with the exception that the left-handed bowler's weight is on the left foot in the stance and the right foot will step out first. Consequently, there is an extra step in the beginning. The ball is still held to the side of the body in the stance but probably a little higher to allow for a little longer arc to take up the extra time of the extra step.

The ball is still pushed out and down in the pushaway after the right foot moves to counteract the weight of the ball. In other words, the bowler takes a small step with the right foot, then moves the ball in the second step. In contrast to the 4-step approach, where the ball starts back on the *second* step, in the 5-step approach, the ball is just starting into the backswing near the *third* step. With the additional length of the swing arc, the small extra step in the beginning should prevent any problems (Figure 12.3).

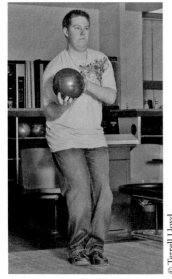

a

© Terrell Lloyd

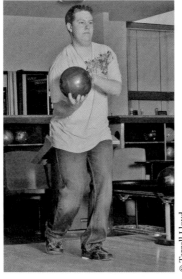

b

© Terrell Lloyd

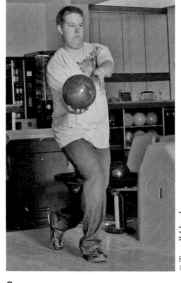

c

© Terrell Lloyd

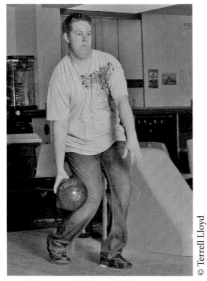

d

© Terrell Lloyd

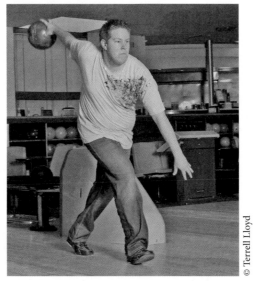

e

© Terrell Lloyd

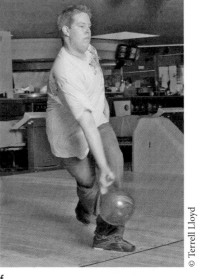

f

© Terrell Lloyd

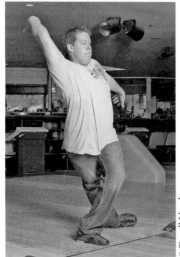

g

© Terrell Lloyd

FIGURE 12.1 A-G A 5-step approach—Right hander.

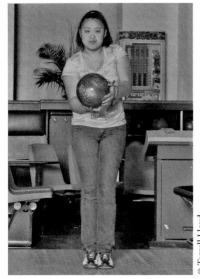

a

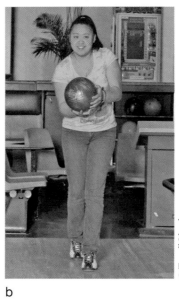

b

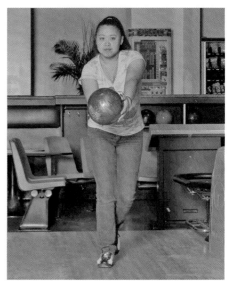

c

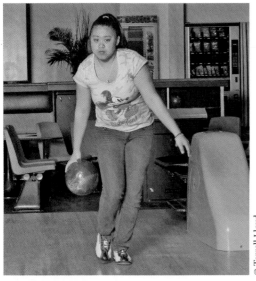

d

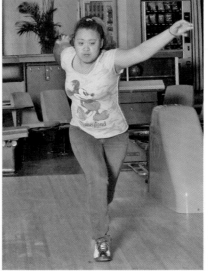

e

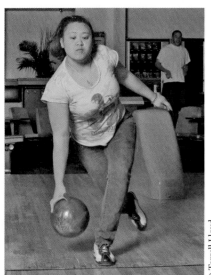

f

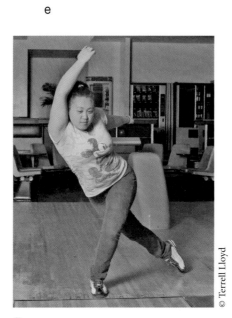

g

FIGURE 12.2 A-G   Front view of 5-step approach

3-Step Approach

It is not an absolute necessity that a **3-step approach** be changed, but if timing problems are resulting from this approach, it is relatively easy to adopt the 4- or 5-step approach with minor adjustments.

The analysis of the timing in the 3-step approach finds the first step of this approach to be the same as the second step in the 4-step for the swing and approach coordination. For right handers, good 3-step timing

should find the ball down by the left leg (first step), ready to go into the backswing of the arc. For left handers, good 3-step timing should find the ball down by the right leg (first step), ready to go into the backswing of the arc. To do this, the bowler must have moved the ball out and down before the feet start the move into the approach. In accordance with the principle of balance we learned previously, the foot should move to maintain balance. But if the foot moves too early in the 3-step approach, the bowler will be out of time. Most 3-step approach bowlers combat this problem by "muscling" the ball to make the swing fit the feet. The resulting steps are usually very large, to give the ball a chance to complete the swing (Figure 12.4).

Maintaining a smooth 3-step approach means that the bowler must eliminate the "muscled" swing and hurried approach, take the stance closer to the foul line, and increase knee flexion to lower the center of gravity.

FIGURE 12.3 A-E A 5-step approach—Left hander.

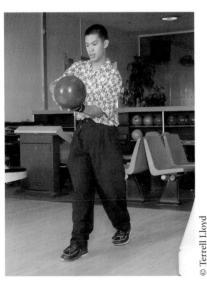

a

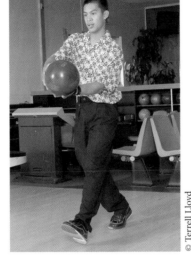

b

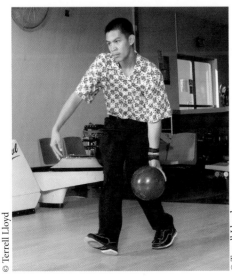

c

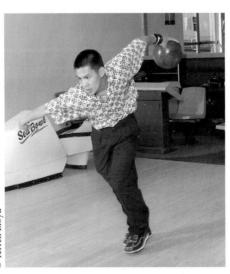

d

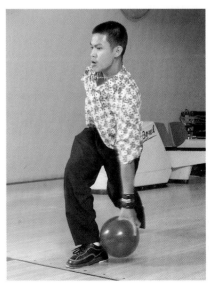

e

No-Step Approach

Many children, senior citizens, and handicapped bowlers have found bowling a challenging and fun activity. Many become good bowlers even though they are unable to take an approach.

We have previously established that both the pendular swing and the approach generate the needed force required on the ball. If a bowler cannot take steps in the approach, more momentum must be generated in the swing. This can be accomplished by holding the ball fairly high in the stance at the foul line, concentrating on keeping the arm and elbow perfectly straight in the swing, and executing a complete follow-through. The follow-through must come up and out at least to eye level and be perfectly straight with the target board or arrow. As always, during the entire swing, absolute concentration is focused on the target board or arrow.

If it is at all possible, a step is advised with the delivery of the ball. Remember to step out and toward your target arrow with the opposite leg of the bowling arm. Try to bend the knee and stay as low as possible to the lane.

A lack of ball speed will result in a greater hook, thereby necessitating adjustments that were discussed in previous sections of this text. The right-handed bowler will probably need to stand left of center, rolling the ball further toward the right. However, the left-handed bowler will probably stand right of center, rolling the ball further toward the left.

Timing for the Advanced Bowler

By definition, timing is a bowler's ability to coordinate the armswing with the footwork. This can be accomplished at various tempos, rhythms, and footwork patterns.

Do not equate the speed of a bowler's footwork with timing. Good timing can be achieved at a great variation of foot speeds. If anything, it is far worse to have slow, deliberate footwork, as no momentum is developed for a natural armswing and a bowler ends up with a muscled swing and inconsistent ball speed.

For an advanced bowler, good timing requires the ball to be at the top of its swing arc at the completion of the next-to-last step (third step of 4-step approach; fourth step of 5-step approach). "Late" timing means that the ball has not reached the top of the arc in time and will arrive at the foul line after the bowler does. This timing error often results in a muscled swing or a "pull" at the release point.

"Early" timing means that the ball has reached the top of the arc too soon and will arrive at the foul line before the bowler does. This timing error often results in a hop, a shuffle step, or a stutter of the footwork in mid-approach. The feet are simply trying to catch up to the armswing.

Timing can be adjusted or corrected most commonly in the pushaway in its relation to the first step. Timing can be adjusted by:

1. Changing when the ball is set in motion.
2. Changing the trajectory or direction of the pushaway.
3. Changing the speed or effort exerted in the pushaway or altering the length of the pushaway.

To Correct "Late" Timing

1. Push the ball away sooner, so that it feels like the ball moves distinctly before the step.
2. Direct the pushaway in a more downward trajectory (i.e., toward the foul line).
3. Increase the effort exerted in the pushaway or accelerate the movement.

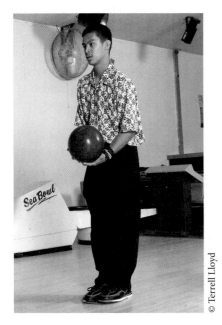

a

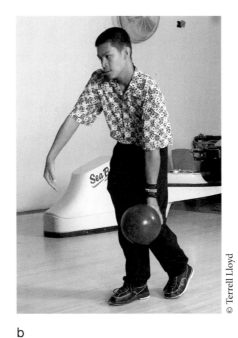

b

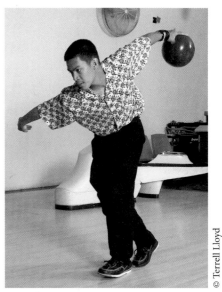

c

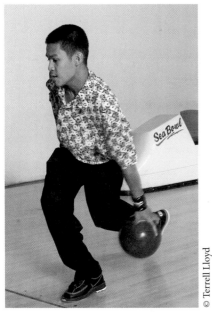

d

FIGURE 12.4 A-D   A 3-step approach.

4. Another alternative might be to lengthen the second step of a 4-step approach (third step of a 5-step approach) to give the ball more time to travel its natural arc.

To Correct "Early" Timing

1. Delay the pushaway, so that it feels like the step takes place before the ball moves away from the body.
2. Direct the pushaway in a more upward trajectory. Visualize a large forward arc into the downswing.
3. Decrease the effort exerted in the pushaway or relax the ball movement.
4. Shorten the second step of a 4-step approach (third step of a 5-step approach) to decrease the length of time the ball has to travel.

In Summary

● Once habits have been formed, they are more difficult to change. Changes usually feel awkward.

- Deviating from the norm in foot and hand position is not uncommon in advanced bowlers.
- The 4-step approach is usually recommended, but bowlers may use others as long as flexibility, balance, and timing are still present.
- The major point to remember in all approaches is that the footwork is adjusted to the swing instead of the swing to the footwork.

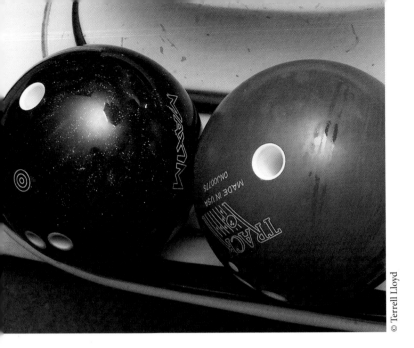

© Terrell Lloyd

13

Ball Tracks

In order to assist advanced bowlers in rolling a more effective ball, it is necessary to identify their particular ball track. The **ball track** is the pattern of "scratch marks" that develop on the surface of the ball. They represent the portion of the ball that touches the lane as it travels toward the pins. This is fairly easy to identify with a bowler who has his or her own ball. Due to the consistent and repetitious release of the ball, a series of nick marks will form on the surface of the ball where it consistently touches the lane. Another method of identifying the track is by observing the oil ring left on the ball or by putting a piece of tape on the ball and watching its rotation pattern as the ball travels down the lane. These wear marks or rotation patterns will usually be indicative of one of the four ball tracks most commonly found in bowling today—the full roller, semi-roller, spinner, and reverse hook (commonly referred to as a backup ball).

It has been stressed throughout this book that the thumb should theoretically (for right handers) be near 10 o'clock at the release point. In actuality, due to the weight of the ball, intended action of the fingers, or a bowler's natural tendencies, the elbow automatically rotates slightly either clockwise or counterclockwise. This is true for right handers and left handers alike. At the release point, a right hander may find the thumb between 9 and 12 o'clock. A left hander may find the thumb between 3 and 12 o'clock.

Identification of Ball Tracks for Right Handers

Full Roller

The **full roller** ball track may be identified by the nick marks passing on the outside of the finger holes and the inside of the thumb hole, splitting the ball in half, thus rolling across the bowler's span. Because it is rolling around 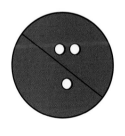 the 27-inch circumference of the ball, it is called a full roller. In a full roller, the thumb rotates in a clockwise direction from 10 to 11 o'clock at the very last instant of thumb release. The fingers lift through and impart a slight counterclockwise rotation on the ball. Thus, there are two rotations being placed on the ball, with the primary rotation being the counter-clockwise one as the fingers release. This slight rotation is a result of the thumb coming out of the ball first and the fingers last. This release method can be an effective one and will often enable the ball to hook slightly from right to left for a right hander. One of the characteristics of a full roller is the fine narrow track on the ball showing great consistency and accuracy, especially on the outside line.

The full roller is an acceptable release because it produces a right-to-left hooking action as the ball travels down the lane, assisting with effective pin action. The full roller also enables a bowler to achieve a consistent and accurate type of release.

Often, it does have trouble carrying strikes because it has an "end over end" roll that results in the ball rolling right through the pin deck, leaving many 4, 7, and 10 pins. It becomes an effective ball when rolled from an outside line. In the twenty-first century, not many bowlers use this type of release method.

Semi-Roller

The second common type of ball track is one where the nick marks pass on the outside of the finger holes and on the outside of the thumb hole. Obviously, this ball is rolling over a smaller portion of the ball instead of the full circumference, so it is called a **semi-roller** or a ¾ **roller.**

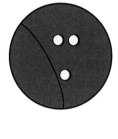

The fingers lift through the ball, also in a counterclockwise direction. The nick marks may vary from being near the thumb hole or as far as 2 inches away.

The advantage of the semi-roller is that it has greater pin action than the other ball rolls because it has a great right-to-left hooking action. The heavier portion of the ball is heading toward the pocket as the ball travels down the lane. Upon pin contact, this heavier portion of the ball will help decrease the ball deflection and will drive the pins sideways, thus increasing the pin carry. Without a consistent approach, this ball roll may lose accuracy because of its increased hooking action. In the twenty-first century, the vast majority of bowlers use this release method.

Spinner

The **spinner** is considered an offshoot of the semi-roller. It is merely an overturned or an exaggerated semi-roller

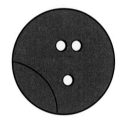

delivery where the thumb rotates too far counter-clockwise, all the way from 11 o'clock toward 8 or 7 o'clock. The ball is actually spinning on a very small portion of the ball surface, reacting like a top going down the lane as it spins on its own axis. Often a spinner can be identified by watching the thumb of the bowler at the release. It will usually be pointing downward (Figure 13.1).

The spinner release travels down the lane in a fairly straight line. As it contacts the pins, it will bounce off in the opposite direction (maximum deflection), similar to the action of a spinning top hitting a wall. As it hits the pocket, it will deflect to the right, leaving spare combinations that include the 5 pin. Due to its straight path, it may be a very effective and accurate ball on very dry lanes when most balls are hooking too much.

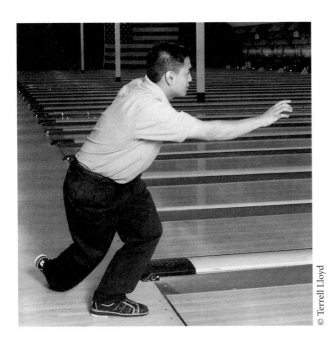

FIGURE 13.1
A spinner is delivered with the palm facing the floor.

© Terrell Lloyd

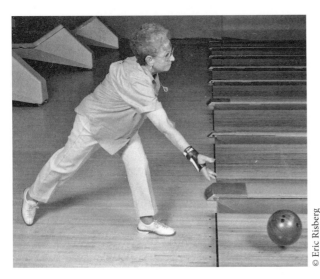

FIGURE 13.2
A backup ball is delivered with the palm facing upward toward the ceiling.

© Eric Risberg

to this exaggeration, the ball cannot receive a counter-clockwise lift with the fingers. Consequently, the fingers continue a clockwise rotation through the release that brings about the left to right or reverse hooking action (Figure 13.2). The backup ball, or reverse hook, is a totally ineffective ball unless the right-handed bowler moves to the left and rolls for the 1-2 pocket. There are three main reasons for this ineffectiveness:

1. It is inconsistent because it is difficult to regulate the excess clockwise rotation placed on the ball.
2. It may put undue strain on the wrist and elbow, causing elbow soreness and tendinitis.
3. It has maximum pin deflection in the 1-3 pocket.

It is also difficult to roll from the left into the Brooklyn side (1-2 pocket) because of the inability to impart enough clockwise rotation and sufficient lift.

Thumper

Even though the thumper is not a recognized type of ball roll, occasionally this track will occur. A **thumper**

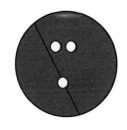

merely finds the ball rolling over the thumb hole down the lane. The thumper is usually caused by insufficient counterclockwise rotation of the fingers at the release point or by the thumb coming out of the thumb hole too early or too late.

To correct this error, the hand position needs to be changed in the stance by moving the thumb and fingers either more to the side of the ball or more underneath the ball (starting at 9 o'clock or 11 o'clock rather than 10 o'clock). The wrist should also be checked to make sure it is firm. If

Backup Ball

The **backup ball,** or **reverse hook,** is basically an offshoot of the full roller. It hooks from left to right, unlike the normal right-left hook for right handers. The thumb rotates clockwise from 10 to 1 or even 2 o'clock, which is an exaggeration of the full roller release. However, due these two suggestions do not work, the ball balance should be checked.

Identification of Ball Tracks for Left Handers

Full Roller

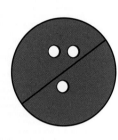

The **full roller** ball track may be identified by the nick marks passing on the outside of the finger holes and the inside of the thumbhole, splitting the ball in half, rolling over the label of the ball. Because it is rolling around the 27-inch circumference of the ball, it is called a full roller. In a full roller, the thumb rotates in a counterclockwise direction from the 2 o'clock to 1 o'clock position at the very last instant of thumb release. The fingers lift through and impart a clockwise rotation on the ball. Thus, there are two rotations being placed on the ball, the primary rotation being the clockwise one as the fingers release. This is a result of the thumb coming out of the ball first and the fingers last. This release method can be a very effective one and will enable the ball to hook from the left to the right for a left hander. One of the characteristics of a full roller is the fine narrow track on the ball showing great consistency and accuracy especially on the outside line.

One of the advantages of the full roller is that it produces a left-to-right hooking action as it travels down the lane, resulting in fairly good pin action. The full roller also enables a bowler to achieve a consistent and accurate type of release.

Often it does have trouble carrying strikes because it has an "end over end" roll that sometimes results in the ball rolling right through the pin deck leaving many 6, 10, and 7 pins. It can become an effective release method when rolled from an outside line.

Semi-Roller

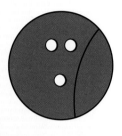

The second common type of ball track is one where the nick marks pass on the outside of the finger holes and on the outside of the thumb hole. Obviously, this ball is rolling over a smaller portion of the ball instead of the full circumference, so it is called a **semi-roller** or a ¾ roller.

The fingers lift through the ball in a clockwise direction. The nick marks may vary from being near the thumb hole or as far as 2 inches away.

The advantage of the semi-roller is that it has greater pin action than the other ball rolls because it has a great left-to-right hooking action. The heavier portion of the ball is heading toward the pocket as the ball travels down the lane. Upon pin contact, this heavier portion of the ball will help decrease the ball deflection and drive the pins sideways, thus increasing the pin carry. Without a consistent approach, this ball roll may lose accuracy because of its increased hooking action. It is likely that at least 95 percent of all left handers use this release method.

Spinner

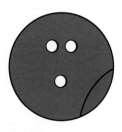

The spinner is considered an offshoot of the semi-roller. It is merely an overturned or exaggerated semi-roller delivery where the thumb rotates too far clockwise, all the way from 1 o'clock toward the 4 or 5 o'clock position. The ball is actually spinning on a very small portion of the ball surface, reacting like a top going down the lane as it spins on its own axis. Often a spinner can be identified by watching the thumb of the bowler at the release. It will usually be pointing downward (Figure 13.1).

The spinner release travels down the lane in a fairly straight line. As it contacts the pins, it will bounce off in the opposite direction (maximum deflection), similar to the action of a spinning top hitting a wall. As it hits the pocket, it will deflect to the left, leaving spare combinations that include the 5 pin. Due to its straight path, it may be a very effective and accurate ball on very dry lanes when most balls are hooking too much.

Backup Ball

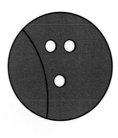

The **backup ball,** or **reverse hook,** is basically an offshoot of the full roller. It hooks from the right to the left unlike the normal left-to-right hook for left handers. The thumb rotates clockwise from 2 to 11 or even 10 o'clock, which is an exaggeration of the full roller release. However, due to this exaggeration, the ball cannot receive a clockwise lift with the fingers. Consequently, the fingers continue a counter-clockwise rotation through the release that brings about the right-to-left or reverse hooking action (Figure 13.2). The backup ball, or reverse hook, is a totally ineffective ball unless the left-handed bowler moves to the right and rolls for the 1-3 pocket. There are three main reasons for this ineffectiveness:

1. It is inconsistent because it is difficult to regulate the excess counter-clockwise rotation placed on the ball.

2. It may put undue strain on the wrist and elbow, causing elbow soreness and tendinitis.

3. It has maximum pin deflection in the 1-2 strike pocket.

It is difficult to roll from the right into the Brooklyn side (1-3 pocket) because of the inability to impart enough counter-clockwise rotation and lift.

Thumper

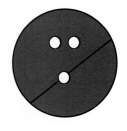

Even though the **thumper** is not a recognized type of ball roll, occasionally this track will occur. A thumper merely finds the ball rolling over the thumb hole all the way down the lane. The thumper is usually caused by insufficient clockwise rotation of the fingers at the release point or by the thumb coming out of the thumb hole too early or too late.

To correct this error, the hand position needs to be changed in the stance by moving the thumb and fingers either more to the side of the ball or more underneath the ball (starting at 3 o'clock or 1 o'clock rather than 2 o'clock). The wrist should also be checked to make sure it is firm. If these two suggestions do not work, the ball balance should be checked.

Corrections and Changes in Ball Tracks for Right Handers

The two most desirable ball tracks are the semi-roller and full roller. It is not a must to change everyone's ball track to one of these two, however. It really depends upon the intention and intensity of the bowler. Many times bowlers can be encouraged to change by showing the disadvantages of the ball they are currently rolling in comparison to the advantages of the full roller or semi-roller. However, change is sometimes painful because the bowler's average will fall and his or her accuracy will definitely diminish during the learning phase.

Backup Ball

We have found that the backup ball (reverse hook) is really an exaggerated full roller. When does a full roller become a backup? Remember, the fingers are lifting counter-clockwise in the full roller but clockwise in the backup. The counter-clockwise rotation in the full roller is caused by the thumb staying left of the 12 o'clock position on the ball at the point of release. Basically, the 12 o'clock position is the cutoff point as to whether the ball becomes a full roller or a backup ball. If the thumb rotates to the 1 or 2 o'clock position, a backup ball will be the result (Figure 13.3).

A backup ball delivery could easily be changed into a full roller, and this may sometimes be accomplished by merely changing the thumb position in the stance from the 10 o'clock position to an 8 or 9 o'clock position. At the point of release, it will be near 12 o'clock, resulting in a full roller rather than the 10 to 2 o'clock rotation, ending in a backup.

Once someone has been convinced to change from the backup ball to a more effective delivery, the following suggestions could be used

FIGURE 13.3 The path of a backup ball for right and left handers (basically, a reverse hook).

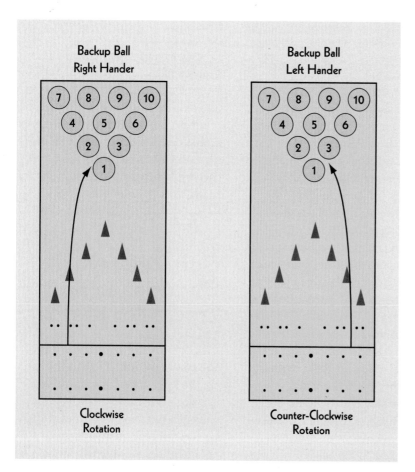

to help in eliminating the backup bowler's habits:

- The bowler is assigned a new target (second arrow from the right) and a new starting position (right arm in line with the target arrow). It all looks and feels wrong to the bowler because he or she feels as though the lane itself is to the left.
- In the stance, the ball should be held off to the right side of the body with the wrist firm. Overemphasize the thumb and finger position by placing them at 9 and 3 o'clock. This exaggeration of hand placement is a teaching gimmick many use to obtain the desired result. This is why the bowler may even be encouraged to place his or her hand at an 8 and 2 o'clock position.
- At the release point, have the bowler execute the follow-through with the index finger (fingernail facing up), pointing toward the target. This automatically puts the thumb in a 9 o'clock position.
- If these suggestions have been tried and the bowler still rolls a backup ball, check the direction of the pushaway. If he or she was used to holding the ball in front of the body rather than to the side, the pushaway probably went out to the right. If he or she continues to do this with the ball held off to the side, the result would be the ball swinging behind his or her back. Anytime the ball swings around the back, there is a tendency to compensate by coming through and rotating the elbow inside out, which results in a backup.
- The next area to check is the knee flexion. If the bowler does not flex the knees and shuffle the feet in the approach, there is a tendency for the shoulder to drop. When the shoulder drops, the elbow rotates.
- If the backup still persists, the rotation of the elbow in the downswing should be checked. In a backup ball, the elbow will rotate inside out. For an exaggerated compensation, the inside of the elbow should be facing the body all of the time, thus placing the thumb at the 9 o'clock position.
- If the wrist rotates at the release point, direct the bowler to point the "V" that is formed by the index finger and thumb toward the target, or to point the index finger at the target as he or she releases the ball.
- The balance of the ball and the pitch of the thumb hole may need to be checked.
- As a last resort, convert the bowler to a semi-roller.

For those bowlers who do not want to change from a backup ball, more effective ball action may be obtained by developing the maximum angle into the pocket. This can be done by adjusting the stance and target arrow so that the bowler is aiming for the 18th board and a "high pocket" hit. The more common advice is to have the ball balanced as if it were drilled for a left hander. This would increase the drive of the ball in the opposite direction as the bowler plays the left side of the lane and aims for the 1-2 pocket.

Full Roller

Many times a bowler rolling a full roller would like to increase the hook on the ball by increasing the lift and side rotation. This can be accomplished by placing the thumb at the 9 o'clock rather than the 10 o'clock position (Figure 13.4). This action will increase the thumb rotation, and therefore increase the counter-rotation of the fingers.

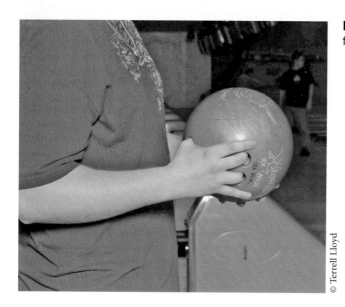

FIGURE 13.4 Hand position for a full roller.

© Terrell Lloyd

The second thing that could be done would be to pull the index finger closer to the gripping fingers and spread the little finger as far out as it will comfortably go. This will help increase the lift on the ball and allow the ball to finish more strongly into the pocket.

Semi-Roller

The changes for a semi-roller are quite opposite to those found in the full roller. Instead of starting with the thumb at 10 o'clock, place it at 12 o'clock with the hand underneath the ball. This will increase the side rotation and lift applied to the ball because of the increased rotation of the fingers at release.

Secondly, the fingers should be adjusted by spreading the index finger out and away from the gripping fingers while pulling the little finger in closer. This action will help to impart a stronger counterclockwise rotation at the release point (Figure 13.5).

In the case of a very slow lane where too much hook is a problem, a bowler could decrease side rotation and hook by simply reversing those actions designed to increase side rotation, as stated in the previous section on the full roller and above on the semi-roller.

Spinner

It is recommended that an effective spinner be converted to a semi-roller because the spinner is an overturned or exaggerated semi-roller. This can easily be accomplished by making sure the wrist is extended and the hand is underneath the weight of the ball. The bowler should attempt to maintain this 2 o'clock position during the release and to keep the elbow straight into the follow-through. This action will ensure the release of the thumb from the thumb hole prior to that of the fingers. The bowler should be reminded that, at the release, he or she should curl the fingers into the palm of the hand with the thumb up.

It is recommended that if someone refuses to change from a spinner, he or she should stand further right and get maximum ball angle upon the entry into the pocket for better pin action and less deflection.

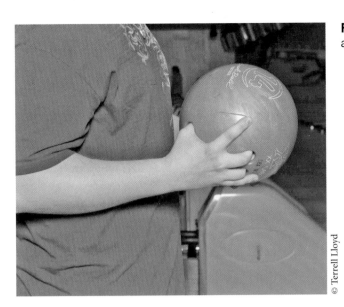

FIGURE 13.5   Hand position for a semi-roller.

© Terrell Lloyd

Corrections and Changes in Ball Tracks for Left Handers

The two most desirable ball tracks are the full roller and the semi-roller. It is not a must to change everyone's ball track to one of these two, however. It really depends upon the intention and intensity of the bowler. Many times, bowlers can be encouraged to change by showing the disadvantages of the ball they are currently rolling in comparison to the advantages of the full roller or semi-roller. However, change is sometimes painful because the bowler's average will fall and his or her accuracy will definitely diminish during the learning phase.

Backup Ball

We have found that the backup ball (reverse hook) is really an exaggerated full roller. When does a full roller become a backup ball? Remember, the fingers are lifting clockwise in the full roller but counter-clockwise in the backup.

Basically, the 12 o'clock position is the cutoff point as to whether the ball becomes a full roller or a backup ball (Figure 13.3).

A backup ball delivery could easily be changed into a full roller, which is sometimes accomplished by merely changing the thumb position in the stance from the 2 o'clock position to a 4 or 3 o'clock position. At the point of release, it will be near 12 o'clock, resulting in a full roller rather than the 2 to 10 o'clock position, ending in a backup.

Once someone has been convinced to change from the backup ball to a more effective delivery, the following suggestions could be used to help in eliminating the backup bowler's habits:

- The bowler is assigned a new target (second arrow from the left) and a new starting position (left arm in line with the target arrow). It all looks and feels wrong to the bowler because he or she feels as though the lane itself is to the right.
- In the stance, the ball should be held off to the left side of the body with the wrist firm. Overemphasize the thumb and finger position

by placing them at 3 and 9 o'clock. This exaggeration of hand placement is a teaching gimmick many use to obtain the desired result. This is why the bowler may even be encouraged to place the hand at a 4 and 10 o'clock position.

- At the release point, have the bowler execute the follow-through with the index finger (fingernail facing up), pointing toward the target. This automatically puts the thumb in a 3 o'clock position.
- If these suggestions have been tried and the bowler still rolls a backup ball, check the direction of the pushaway. If he or she was used to holding the ball in front of the body rather than to the side, the pushaway probably went out to the left. If he or she continues to do this with the ball held off to the side, the result would be the ball swinging behind his or her back. Anytime the ball swings around the back, there is a tendency to compensate by coming through and rotating the elbow inside out, which results in a backup.
- The next area to check is the knee flexion. If the bowler does not flex the knees and shuffle the feet in the approach, there is a tendency for the shoulder to drop. When the shoulder drops, the elbow rotates.
- If the backup still persists, the rotation of the elbow in the downswing should be checked. In a backup ball, the elbow will rotate inside out. For an exaggerated compensation, the inside of the elbow should be facing the body all of the time, thus placing the thumb at the 3 o'clock position.
- If the wrist rotates at the release point, direct the bowler to point the "V" that is formed by the index finger and thumb toward the target, or to point the index finger at the target as he or she releases the ball.

- The balance of the ball and the pitch of the thumb hole might need to be checked.
- As a last resort, convert the bowler to a semi-roller.

For those bowlers who do not want to change from a backup ball, more effective ball action may be obtained by developing maximum angle into the pocket. This can be done by adjusting the stance and target arrow so that the bowler is aiming high for the 18th board and a "high pocket" hit. The more common advice is to have the ball balanced as if it were drilled for a right hander. This would increase the drive of the ball in the opposite direction as the bowler plays the right side of the lane and aims for the 1-3 pocket.

Full Roller

Many times a bowler rolling a full roller would like to increase the hook on the ball by increasing the lift and side rotation. This can be accomplished by placing the thumb at the 3 o'clock rather than the 2 o'clock position (Figure 13.4). This action will increase the thumb rotation, and, therefore, increase the counter-rotation of the fingers.

The second thing that could be done would be to pull the index finger closer to the gripping fingers and spread the little finger as far out as it will comfortably go. This will help increase the lift on the ball and will allow the ball to finish more strongly into the pocket.

Semi-Roller

The changes for a semi-roller are quite opposite to those found in the full roller. Instead of starting with the thumb at 2 o'clock, place it at 12 o'clock with the hand underneath the ball. This will increase the side rotation and lift applied to the ball because of the increased rotation of the fingers at release.

Secondly, the fingers should be adjusted by spreading the index finger in closer. This action will help to impart a stronger clockwise rotation at the release point (Figure 13.5).

In the case of a very slow lane where too much hook is a problem, a bowler could decrease side rotation and hook by simply reversing those actions designed to increase side rotation, as stated in the previous section on the full roller and above on the semi-roller.

Spinner

It is recommended that an effective spinner be converted to a semi-roller because the spinner is an overturned or exaggerated semi-roller. This can easily be accomplished by making sure the wrist is extended and the hand is underneath the weight of the ball. The bowler should attempt to maintain this 10 o'clock position during the release and to keep the elbow straight into the follow-through. This action will ensure the release of the thumb from the thumb hole prior to that of the fingers. The bowler should be reminded that at the release, he or she should curl the fingers into the palm of the hand with the thumb up. It is recommended that if someone refuses to change from a spinner, he or she should stand further left and get maximum angle upon the entry into the pocket for better pin action and less deflection.

Hints for Success:

- For **right handers to correct a spinner,** start with the thumb at 12 or 1 o'clock. Concentrate on keeping the elbow close to the hip during the swing and attempt to release the ball with the thumb at 12 o'clock (an over-exaggeration). Also, try to keep the inside of the elbow facing forward toward the pins and avoid allowing the elbow to flex early and bend outward at the release. Visualize attempting to roll a straight or backup ball. This will result in a semi-roller.

- For **left handers to correct a spinner,** start with the thumb at 11 or 12 o'clock. Concentrate on keeping the elbow close to the hip during the swing and attempt to release the ball with the thumb at 12 o'clock (an over-exaggeration). Also, try to keep the inside of the elbow facing forward toward the pins and avoid allowing the elbow to flex early and bend outward at the release. Visualize attempting to roll a straight or backup ball. This will result in a semi-roller.

- **To create a full roller from a backup ball, right handers** start the thumb at 8 or 9 o'clock. During the swing, keep the inside of the elbow facing toward the body to keep the thumb in a downward position throughout the swing. At the release, direct the index finger toward the target.

- **To create a full roller from a backup ball, left handers** start the thumb at 4 or 3 o'clock. During the swing, keep the inside of the elbow facing toward the body to keep the thumb in a downward position throughout the swing. At the release, direct the index finger toward the target.

In Summary

Changes should be made in the ball tracks only when the ball track presently rolled has been properly identified. The prescription changes are unique to each ball roll pattern. Methods of identifying ball tracks include:

- By the nick marks scarred into the ball surface.
- By the oil ring left on the ball (Figure 13.6).
- By putting a tracer on the ball in the center of the span and watching its action (Figure 13.7).

1. In a full roller, this tracer would roll very high and end over end while angled to the left.
2. In a semi-roller, it would roll in a much tighter circle on the left.
3. In a spinner, it would be in a very tiny compact roll or going around in a Saturn-type ring, or almost stationary on top of the ball.
4. In a backup, the tracer would be rolling on the right side of the ball.

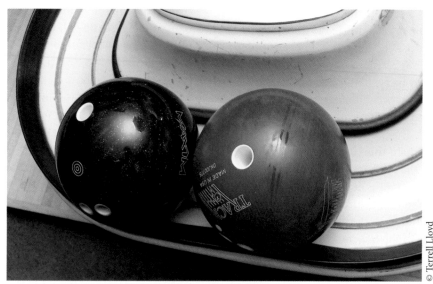

FIGURE 13.6
The oil ring and wear marks are evident on these two bowling balls.

© Terrell Lloyd

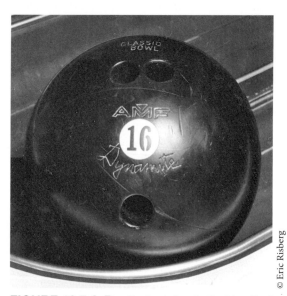

© Eric Risberg

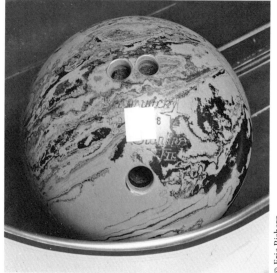

© Eric Risberg

FIGURE 13.7 A-B   On the left, a ball with a "built-in" tracer denoting the ball's weight. On the right, a ball with a piece of white tape placed in the center of the span.

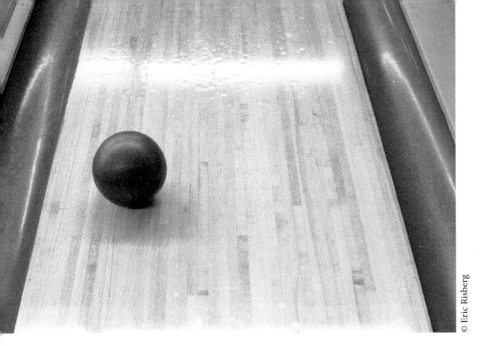
© Eric Risberg

14

Lift and Revolutions

Previously, we learned that the ball is most effective when it travels at an average speed of 17 miles per hour with the right amount of forward roll and side rotation. **Lift,** which is imparted on the ball at the release, produces the forward revolutions and accentuates the side rotation on the ball. Lift is the pressure a bowler feels on his or her fingertips at the release point after the thumb has been removed from the ball. It is the resistance created when the weight of the ball, which is a downward force, meets the resistance of the fingers moving in an upward direction. The action of the thumb and fingers at the release finds the thumb coming out at the bottom of the swing and the fingers remaining for a split second longer into the upswing phase of the arc. This is the point at which lift creating revolutions ("revs") is developed and felt.

Lift

Because it is nearly impossible to practice lift by itself, several conscious acts can be practiced to get lift to happen more automatically and consistently:

- The body should arrive at the foul line a split second before the ball. This will put the body in a "set" position and the ball can come through with maximum leverage on the hand underneath the weight of the ball.
- The vertical balance line must be perfectly positioned over the bent forward knee in order to impart effective lift on the ball (Figure 14.1). In any other position, the hand will not be underneath the weight of the ball.
- A good horizontal balance line must be achieved by counter-balancing the weight of the ball on the right with the extension of body parts on the left (right handers). Left handers have a good horizontal balance line when the weight of the ball on the left is balanced with the extension of the body parts on the right.
- The ball must be as close as possible to the forward ankle to impart lift. This distance is usually about 2 to 4 inches from the outside of the ball because it would be quite difficult to impart lift on an object 2 feet away from the vertical line of the body (refer to Figure 14.2).
- The last step must be varied a bit from the norm by stepping slightly into the ball path. This brings the ball closer to the forward ankle.

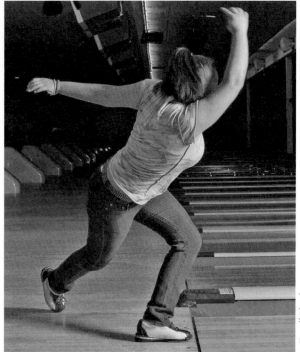

a

© Terrell Lloyd

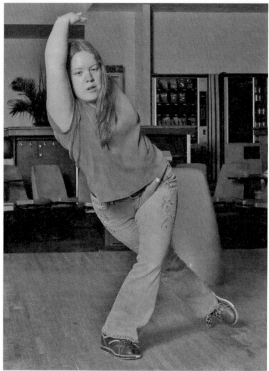

b

© Terrell Lloyd

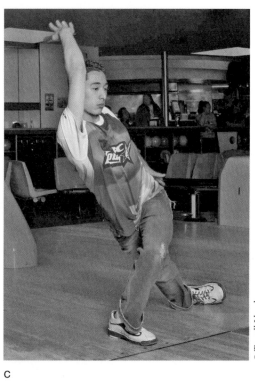

c

© Terrell Lloyd

FIGURE 14.1 A-C   To have leverage in order to apply lift, the slide knee must be bent.

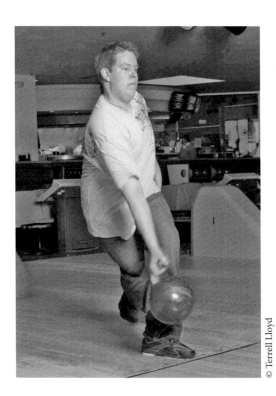

FIGURE 14.2 Lift occurs after the thumb comes out of the ball.

© Terrell Lloyd

- The bowling ball must fit properly in terms of span and hole sizes for the bowler to feel the ball's weight against the hand.

At the release, it is a necessity to get the maximum "feel" of the ball. Three suggestions are given here on how to increase this control factor:

- Concentrate on obtaining a feeling of the ball rolling off the hand.
- Practice squeezing the ball with the fingers while relaxing the thumb at the point of release.
- Curl the fingers into the palm of the hand at the release (Figure 14.3).

Revolutions

For right handers, the product of lift is counter-clockwise **revolutions** or turns of the ball. For left handers, the lift will produce clockwise revolutions. This is due to the application of the lifting pressure off the ball's center of gravity. An effective ball roll will have at least 10 to 12 revolutions as it travels toward the pins. It is possible to achieve more revolutions without compensating in the delivery. The closer a bowler can get to a greater number of revolutions while maintaining speed, the more effective the ball becomes (Figure 14.4).

Please note: The advanced bowlers today have a new common term of "Rev Rate"—Revolutions per minute. Because "Rev Rate" is directly related to ball speed and pin action, the better bowler is constantly working different formulas (check internet) to calculate one's "Rev Rate." Even though there is no "perfect" rev rate for all bowlers, there are different ways of measuring and finding deficiencies in rev rate that affects strong (or weak) pin carry.

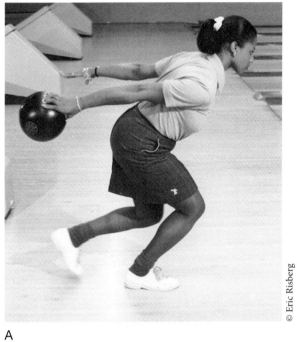

A

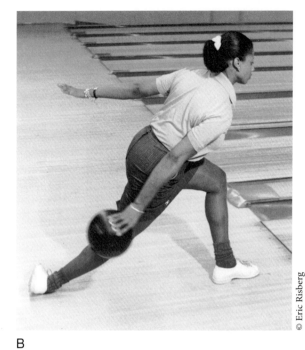

B

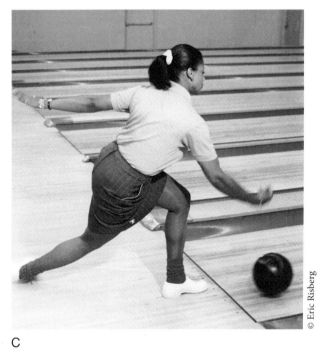

C

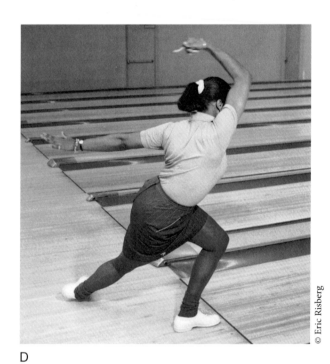

D

FIGURE 14.3 A-D   To apply lift, the knees remain flexed throughout the delivery, the balance line is maintained, and the wrist and fingers remain firm.

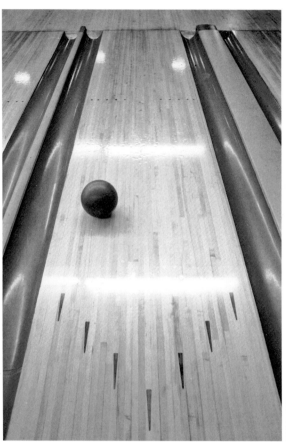

© Eric Risberg

FIGURE 14.4 The ball is most effective when it travels down the lane at an average speed of 17 miles per hour with the right amount of forward roll and side rotation.

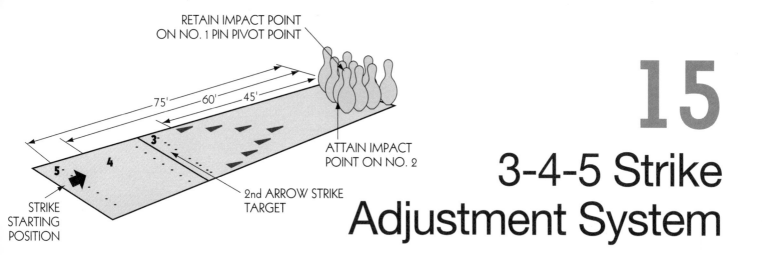

RETAIN IMPACT POINT
ON NO. 1 PIN PIVOT POINT

75'   60'   45'

3

4

5

STRIKE
STARTING
POSITION

ATTAIN IMPACT
POINT ON NO. 2

2nd ARROW STRIKE
TARGET

15
3-4-5 Strike
Adjustment System

The 3-4-5 strike adjustment system is used by the more advanced bowler who has the ability to aim for and hit a specific board on the lane. This strike adjustment is used when the bowler is experiencing difficulty in "carrying" strikes even though the ball is entering the pocket. The aim is accurate but the missing ingredient is the appropriate angle of entry into the pocket. This 3-4-5 strike adjustment system will increase or decrease the angle into the pocket.

In this system, the **pivot point** or constant is the pocket, because the bowler has already established the correct impact point on the head pin but is seeking the correct impact point on the 3 pin. In adjusting for a better angle of entry, the bowler must make a change in the starting position and the target. Both the starting position and the target will be moved at the same time and in the same direction.

The proportions for the 3-4-5 adjustment are: **for every 5 boards the feet are moved in the stance, the target is moved 3 boards.** Again, using a mathematical ratio, this system will work across the lane in either direction as long as the movement is 5 boards for the stance and 3 boards

for the target. Remember, it is 75 feet from the third row of locator dots, 45 feet from the targets, and 60 feet from the foul line to the head pin. The ratio of the locator dots and the target arrows in relation to the total length of the lane is 5:3 (Figures 15.1 and 15.2).

For right handers, the following guidelines should be used in implementing the 3-4-5 system. If the ball is entering the pocket heavy or at too much angle, adjust left. If you are hitting light in the pocket or at too little angle, move right. If the pin leaves consistently involve the 4 pin, or the 4-7 and 4-9 combinations, the ball is driving through the pocket too strongly, so the adjustment would be toward the left. Specifically, the move would be 5 boards to the left in the stance and 3 boards to the left with the target. The results will be the ball hitting the pocket at a decreased (flatter) angle.

If the ball enters the pocket but is consistently leaving the 5 pin, 5-7, 8-10, or 2-4-5 pin combinations, the reverse situation is occurring. The ball is hitting the pocket light with too little angle. The adjustment would be to move the starting position 5 boards to the right. The result will be the ball entering the pocket with a greater angle.

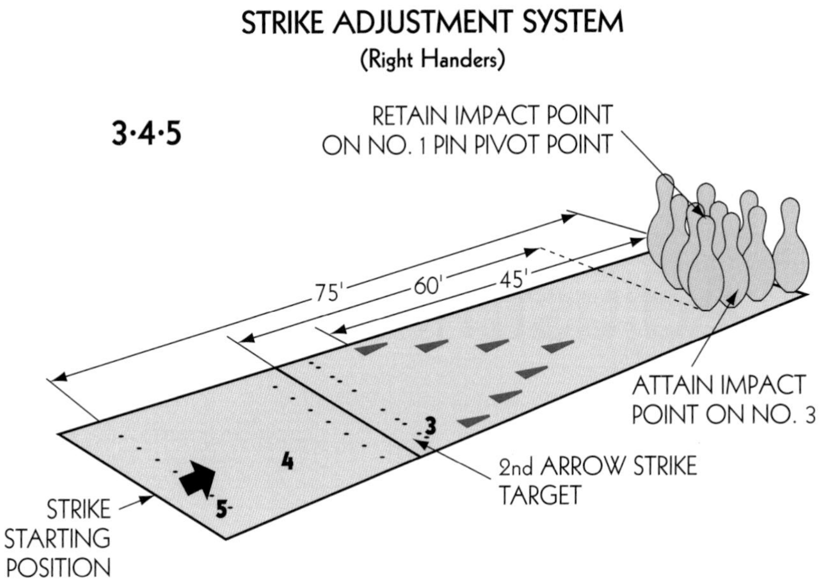

STRIKE ADJUSTMENT SYSTEM
(Right Handers)

3·4·5

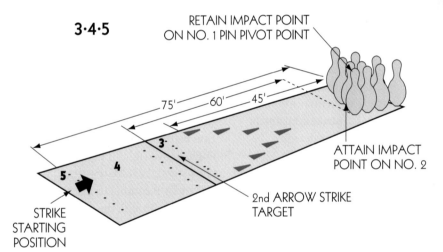

RETAIN IMPACT POINT
ON NO. 1 PIN PIVOT POINT

75'   60'   45'

ATTAIN IMPACT
POINT ON NO. 3

3

4

2nd ARROW STRIKE
TARGET

STRIKE
STARTING
POSITION

5-

FIGURE 15.1   The 3-4-5 Strike Adjustment System for right handers. (Courtesy of former NBC)

STRIKE ADJUSTMENT SYSTEM
(Left Handers)

3·4·5

RETAIN IMPACT POINT
ON NO. 1 PIN PIVOT POINT

75'   60'   45'

3

4

5

ATTAIN IMPACT
POINT ON NO. 2

2nd ARROW STRIKE
TARGET

STRIKE
STARTING
POSITION

FIGURE 15.2   The 3-4-5 Strike Adjustment System for left handers. (Courtesy of former NBC)

For left handers, the following guidelines should be used in implementing the 3-4-5 system. If the ball is entering the pocket heavy or at too much angle, adjust right. If you are hitting light in the pocket or at too little angle, move left. If the pin leaves consistently involve the 6 pin or the 6-10 and 6-8 combinations, the ball is driving through the pocket too strongly, so the adjustment would be toward the right. Specifically, the move would be 5 boards to the right

in the stance and 3 boards to the right with the target. The results will be the ball hitting the pocket at a decreased or flatter angle.

If the ball enters the pocket but is consistently leaving the 5 pin, 5-10, 9-7, or 3-5-6 pin combinations, the reverse situation is occurring. The ball is hitting the pocket light with too little angle. The adjustment would be to move the starting position 5 boards to the left. The result will be the ball entering the pocket with a greater angle.

If the adjustment is insufficient and the situation continues, a good bowler will keep moving and adjusting. The ball will still contact the 1-3 pocket (1-2 pocket, lefties), but the entry will be at a different angle.

This system should work regardless of the target that is being used for the strike line and because the mathematical makeup will work in any proportion. It can be doubled (10:6) for a larger adjustment or cut in half (2.5:1.5) for minor adjustment.

In Summary

- The 3-4-5 system is used by advanced bowlers who are consistently hitting the pocket but not carrying strikes.
- This system merely changes the bowling ball's angle of entry into the pocket without affecting the accuracy.
- The pivot point is the pocket, making it necessary to make two adjustments—one with the feet and the other with the target.
- The rules governing this mathematical ratio are:
  1. For every 5 boards the feet move, the target is moved 3 boards.
  2. Both the feet and the target move in the same direction.
  3. If the ball is hitting heavy, right handers move left. Left handers move right.
  4. If the ball is hitting light, right handers move right. Left handers move left.
- The 5:3 ratio may be doubled or cut in half and used successfully because it is mathematically based.
- The system will work regardless of what strike line is used, and will not break down regardless of the number of moves.
- **Remember,** once an adjustment is made, the bowler must turn the body and the feet to face and walk toward the target.

Self Evaluation QUESTIONS?

1. If a bowler is using the second arrow as the strike target but is leaving the following pins, what adjustment should be made?
   a. 4 pin
   b. 5 pin
   c. 5-7
   d. 4-7

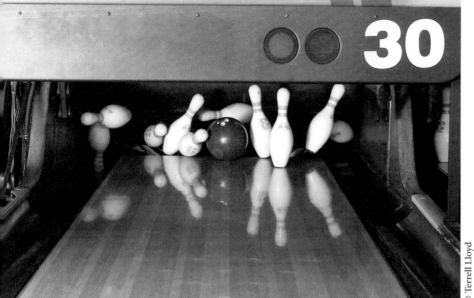
© Terrell Lloyd

16

2-4-6 Spare Adjustment System

Advanced bowlers often adopt the **2-4-6 spare adjustment system** instead of the 3-6-9 system, especially when playing an inside or outside strike line. For a right-handed bowler, **playing an inside line** means that the bowler is using a strike target to the left of the second arrow; playing to the right of the second arrow would be an outside line. For the left-handed bowler, playing an inside line means that the bowler is using a strike target to the right of the second arrow; playing to the left of the second arrow would be an outside line. The 3-6-9 system is of greater advantage for beginners, whose target is basically the second arrow or somewhere between the 8th and 12th board. However, it does have limitations and starts to break down if the target moves from this area. To use this system, the bowler must have developed enough accuracy and consistency so that he or she can adjust and hit a specific board rather than a large target arrow, because the target board will change. Instead of the pivot point or constant being the target arrow, the constant now becomes the stance position of the bowler. The bowler will have two starting positions on the approach when using the 2-4-6 system. **For right handers,** one will be the strike position, which will

be used for all spares standing in the center and on the left side of the lane. The second starting position (10-pin starting position) will be established for rolling at pins on the right side of the lane.

For left handers, the two starting positions will be the strike position, used for all spares standing in the center and on the right side of the lane, and the 7-pin starting position, for picking up spares on the left side of the lane. These starting positions will remain constant in this adjustment system. Instead of moving the starting position as in the 3-6-9 system, the bowler is now going to shift the target.

The basic rule of thumb for the 2-4-6 system states that when a spare adjustment is necessary, **for right handers the spare target will be moved left of the strike target in increments of 2 boards** (Figures 16.1 and 16.2).

For left handers, the spare target will be moved right of the strike target in increments of 2 boards.

For Right Handers

For all spares in the center where the key pin is the 1 or the 5 pin, the bowler stands in the strike starting position

149

and rolls over the strike board or target.

For all spares on the left (2, 4, 7, or 8 pins), the stance is still the strike starting position but the target will shift to the left 2 boards for each pin to the left of the head pin. If the bowler leaves any spare combinations where the key pin is the 2 pin, the bowler will stand in the strike position. To use the second arrow as the target (10th board), the bowler would move the target 2 boards to the left (12th board). However, if the bowler leaves a 4 pin, he or she will stay in the same strike starting position but roll the ball 4 boards to the left of the strike board (14th board). If the key pin is the 7 pin, the bowler would move the target 6 boards left of the strike board (16th board). See Figure 16.1.

The only way the spare and strike systems will work consistently is if the bowler points the toes toward the key pin and walks toward that key pin and the target. If this rule is followed, the 2-4-6 spare adjustment system will work regardless of which board is used as the strike target.

For all spares on the right, as in the 3-6-9 system, the bowler must find the 10-pin starting position through trial and error. It should be noted that if the bowler has been using the 3-6-9 system, this would be the same starting position. In searching for the exact 10-pin starting location, the third arrow should always be used for the target arrow. The basic rule still applies, which is that you start from the left to roll for pins on the right.

SPARE ADJUSTMENT SYSTEM
(Right Handers)

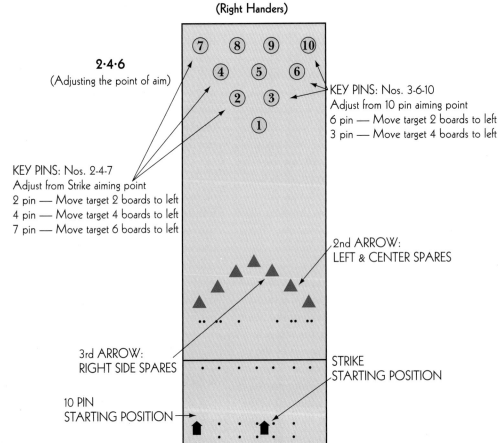

2·4·6
(Adjusting the point of aim)

KEY PINS: Nos. 3-6-10
Adjust from 10 pin aiming point
6 pin — Move target 2 boards to left
3 pin — Move target 4 boards to left

KEY PINS: Nos. 2-4-7
Adjust from Strike aiming point
2 pin — Move target 2 boards to left
4 pin — Move target 4 boards to left
7 pin — Move target 6 boards to left

2nd ARROW:
LEFT & CENTER SPARES

3rd ARROW:
RIGHT SIDE SPARES

STRIKE
STARTING POSITION

10 PIN
STARTING POSITION

FIGURE 16.1 The 2-4-6 Spare Adjustment System for right-handed bowlers. (Courtesy of former NBC)

After the 10-pin starting position has been determined, it will be used for all right side spares. If the 6 pin is left, the target is moved 2 boards to the left of the third arrow (17th board). To pick up the 3 or 9 pin from this same starting position, move the target 4 boards to the left of the third arrow (19th board).

It is a must to find the strike target, the strike starting position, and the 10-pin starting position before one can use this system effectively. This may explain why professional bowlers may sometimes bowl from the extreme right (an outside line) and other times from the left (an inside line). More than likely he or she has established a different strike line or target due to the lane conditions and is using this spare conversion system.

For Left Handers

For all spares on the right (3-6-9-10), the stance is still the strike starting position but the target will shift to the right 2 boards for each pin to the right of the head pin. If the bowler leaves any spare combinations where the key pin is the 3 pin, the bowler will stand in the strike position and, to use the second arrow as the target (10th board), the bowler would move the target two boards to the right (12th board). However, if the bowler leaves the 6 pin, he or she will stay in the same strike starting position but roll the ball four boards to the right of the strike board (14th board). If the key pin is the 10 pin, the bowler would move the target 6 boards right of the strike board (16th board). See Figure 16.2.

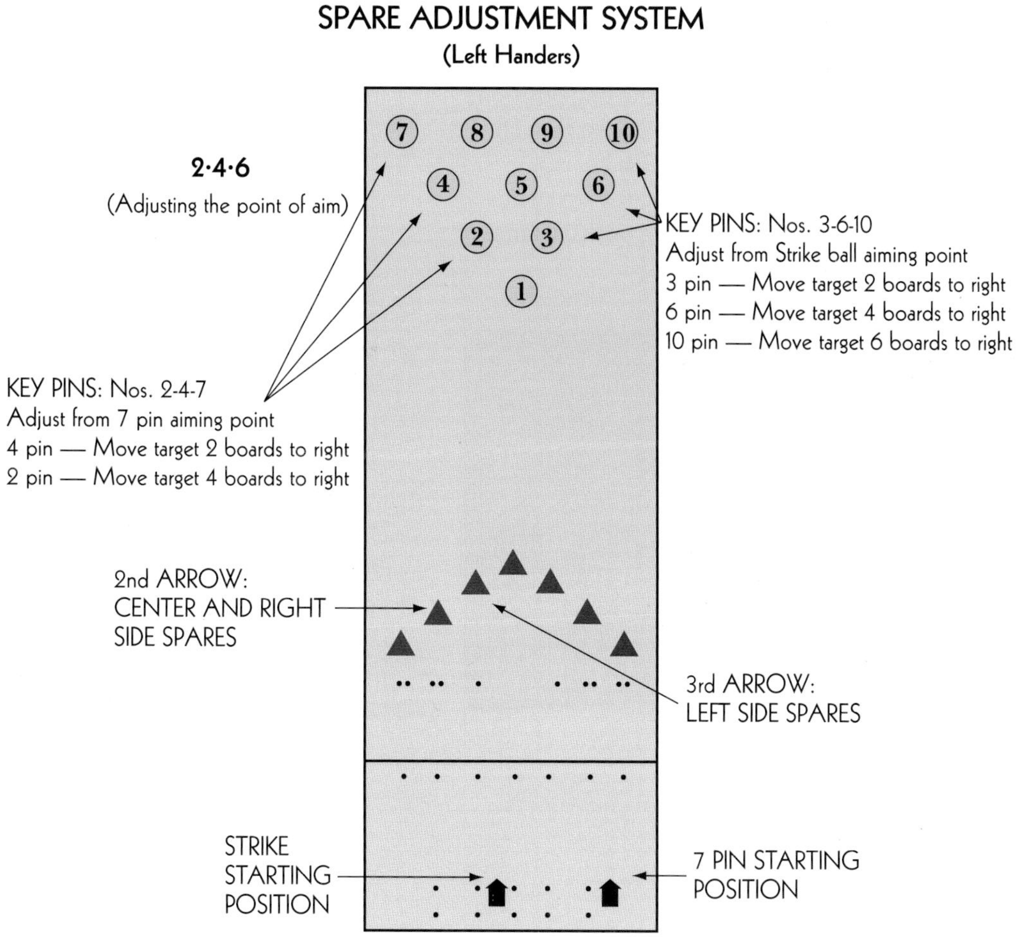

SPARE ADJUSTMENT SYSTEM
(Left Handers)

2·4·6
(Adjusting the point of aim)

KEY PINS: Nos. 3-6-10
Adjust from Strike ball aiming point
3 pin — Move target 2 boards to right
6 pin — Move target 4 boards to right
10 pin — Move target 6 boards to right

KEY PINS: Nos. 2-4-7
Adjust from 7 pin aiming point
4 pin — Move target 2 boards to right
2 pin — Move target 4 boards to right

2nd ARROW: CENTER AND RIGHT SIDE SPARES

3rd ARROW: LEFT SIDE SPARES

STRIKE STARTING POSITION

7 PIN STARTING POSITION

FIGURE 16.2 The 2-4-6 Spare Adjustment System for left-handed bowlers. (Courtesy of former NBC)

The only way the spare and strike systems will work consistently is if the bowler points the toes toward the key pin and walks toward that key pin and the target. If this rule is followed, the 2-4-6 spare adjustment system will work regardless of which board is used as the strike target.

For all spares on the left (2-4-7-8), as in the 3-6-9 spare adjustment system, the bowler must find the 7-pin starting position through trial and error. It should be noted that if the bowler has been using the 3-6-9 system, this would be the same starting position. In searching for the exact 7-pin starting location, the third arrow should always be used for the target arrow. The basic rule still applies, which is that you start from the right to roll for pins on the left.

After the 7-pin starting position has been determined, it will be used for all left-side spares. If the 4 pin is left standing, the target is moved 2 boards to the right of the third arrow (17th board). To pick up the 2 and 8 pins from this same starting position, move the target 4 boards to the right of the third arrow (19th board).

It is a must to find the strike target, the strike starting position, and the 7-pin starting position (10 pin for lefties) before one can use this system effectively. This may explain why professional bowlers may sometimes bowl from the extreme left (an outside line). More than likely the bowler has established a different strike line or target due to the lane conditions and is using this spare conversion system.

In Summary

- When using the 2-4-6 spare conversion system, the two starting positions become the pivot points. The target is moved in increments of 2 boards to the left in accordance with the key pin. (For left handers, the target always moves to the right.)
- This system is used by those who have a consistent approach and can place the ball over specific target boards.
- This system is used by the more advanced bowlers who may vary the strike line to take advantage of specific lane conditions.
- For right-handed bowlers, there are two starting positions in the stance: the strike starting position, used for center and left-side spares, and the 10-pin starting position, used in converting pins on the right.
- For left-handed bowlers, there are also two starting positions in the stance: the strike starting position, used for center and right-side spares, and the 7-pin starting position, used in converting pins on the left.
- At all times when using this system, the stance and approach are always angled toward the key pin or target board.

Self Evaluation QUESTIONS?

1. In order to pick up the following pins, at which board will the bowler aim?

   a. 10 pin

   b. 6 pin

   c. 3 pin

   d. 9 pin

   e. 3-6-7

   f. 6-9

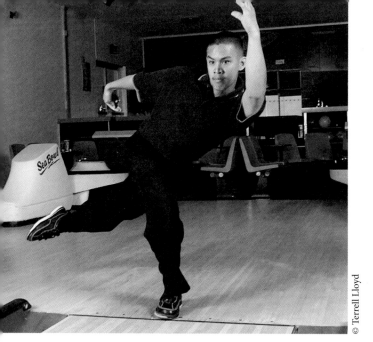

© Terrell Lloyd

17

The Advanced Bowler and Technology

The advanced modern bowler is finding a whole new bowling world with the advent of technology. Chapter 11 gave an overview of some of the technological changes that are taking place in bowling—some being in the equipment (balls, lanes, oiling, or dressing), and some being in the way different ability groups now compete. All of these changes have profoundly affected the way the modern advanced bowler selects the ball and equipment, delivers the ball, aims, and makes adjustments for lane conditions. It is the intent of this chapter to give an overview of some of the adjustments that may be employed by the modern advanced bowler.

Lanes and Lane Condition Adjustments

Because most of the new lanes that are being installed are laminated synthetic lanes and the oiling or dressing amounts and patterns are regulated via computer-type programs, many bowlers are finding that the lanes have a different "feel" from the wooden lanes of the past. Some of the bowlers feel that the general effect of the new oiling patterns and

requirements result in an oilier lane where the ball does not hook as much. Others may feel that their ball hooks more "strongly" in the "back end." To assist the modern bowler, 2 dark boards (each about 3 feet long) have been added about two-thirds of the way down the lane (or about 40 feet). The purpose of these additional targets is to assist the modern player in judging the "break point" (the point where the ball stops sliding and starts its move to the pins—usually the farthest point from the pins in the ball path) (Figure 11.1). This break point is also referred to as the fulcrum point. The modern advanced bowler is very concerned with playing the break point, some 40–45 feet down the lane. Finding this break point and then playing it to ensure the best entry into the pins is of utmost importance. There are a number of ways the advanced player will try to find the perfect break point:

1. A bowler will read the lane to:
   a. Find where the oil is in the front ("head") of the lane.
   b. Find where the dry part of the lane is in relation to the gutter so as to determine how far "out" (toward the gutter) the ball can be rolled.
   c. Find how far "down" the lane the oil is placed.

153

2. Find the break point by:
   a. Altering loft distance out into the lane.
   b. Altering the ball speed, which many find very difficult to regulate.

The adjustments to find the break point are made in the starting position (point of origin) and the target. These adjustments are much greater in modern-day bowling than in the past. A bowler actually has to move a minimum of 3 boards with the feet in the starting position to make any real change in the ball's path. The most common adjustment used today is to adjust "3-2 left." The 3-2 left is performed by moving the feet in the starting position 3 boards to the left and then adjusting the target 2 boards left. This is done on a recreational lane as the oil pattern on the lane (usually a Christmas Tree or a Top Hat) "breaks down." If anyone was observing three different bowlers making their adjustments, they would find three bowlers with varying degrees of hook rolling the ball across the second, third, and fourth arrows, all trying to find the same break point which is common to all three players at the 40-45 foot distance.

The modern-day advanced bowler needs to be very adept in adjusting to lane conditions. It is paramount in tournament play to be able to make these quick "reads" and adjustments. Lane conditions vary from pair to pair, lane to lane, and minute to minute.

Spare Shooting

The first spare adjustment a modern player will use to pick up spares is to use a plastic (polyester) ball. The idea is to take the lane dressing "out of play" when converting spares. Spare shooting requires accuracy rather than hook and power. Bowlers may use more than one ball while competing in bowling.

The second adjustment the modern player would make to pick up spares is to use the 3-6-9 spare conversion system or a modified version thereof. Commonly, a modern right-handed player uses the 3-6-9 system for leftside spares, and will use the 4-8-12 system for spares on the right. The 4-8-12 adjustment shifts the target one-half arrow to the left and moves the feet to the left of the strike starting position either 4, 8, or 12 boards.

Bowling Balls

The newest trend in bowling balls is the reactive resin ball which has an additive that can be sanded or polished to the needs of the user. This ball reacts very well on the new oiling patterns placed on today's lanes. This ball comes with a core that can be either symmetrical or asymmetrical, which ultimately affects the way the ball will react on the lane and against the pins. To assure the bowler that the ball is drilled properly and to each ball's specifications, a knowledgeable, certified professional ball driller needs to be used. *Remember:* In general, a bowling ball can only be drilled to the maximum potential of that bowling ball's characteristics. The *way* that it is drilled can only create a maximum of a 4-6 inch difference in a hook/roll pattern. But changing the surface of the ball through sanding or polishing can change the hook/roll pattern of the ball by feet, not just inches.

The other characteristic in modern-day ball construction affects the radius of the gyration as the ball travels down the lane. There are two basic types of ball construction that deal with gyration—the center heavy and cover heavy. The center heavy ball has a low radius of gyration (RG) allowing the ball to go into a roll more easily. It has a tendency to create a "curve" pattern going down the lane. The second type, the cover heavy, is a ball that has a high RG and is harder to get into a roll. It has a tendency to go farther down the lane before "snapping" (or going into the hook), which creates a sharper, more dramatic hook.

Before you select a new ball for the new century, it is advised that you try out balls with different cores, surfaces, and constructions to get a feel for what is desirable for you. For a guideline in terms of the priorities used to determine your choice of equipment, the priorities are as follows (with influence rating):

1. Type of ball (i.e., plastic, urethane, resin, resin w/additive) 100 pts.
2. Surface of ball (i.e., shiny, dull, in-between)10 pts.
3. Internal dynamics of ball (i.e., cover or center heavy) 1 pt.
4. Static weights (i.e., top, side, finger, and thumb weights) .001 pt.

"Sport Bowling"

In Chapter 11 we explained the new trend of "sport bowling" and how this competition takes place on lanes with sophisticated oiling patterns. This new program consists of advanced players who desire a greater challenge in the game of bowling and are required to do more "shot-making" than needed in the recreational leagues. Absolute control of one's game is required. The recreational bowler playing on the sport bowling conditions could expect a pin drop of 20-25 in average. If a sport bowler has established an average on sport bowling lanes, the USBC has created a chart (Figure 11.2) for this bowler to determine an equivalent average for recreational bowling. For those with an interest in this type of competition, leagues are being formed throughout the United States that will bowl on sport bowling lane conditions.

Approach Characteristics of an Advanced Modern Player

If a person happens to be watching the professionals in a bowling tournament, whether in person or on television, probably the first thing that is noticed is the variety of approach and delivery styles of these men and women. With the advent of the new balls and the sophistication in lane conditions, we also find that many of the bowlers are straying from the traditional method of approach, delivery, and aiming. Some of the things that you may witness will be:

1. The modern player tends to have an "open shoulder" swing to create more energy with less muscle (Figure 17.1). The shoulder will close (or square

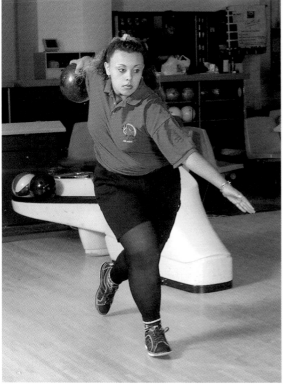

FIGURE 17.1 Open shoulder swing.

© Terrell Lloyd

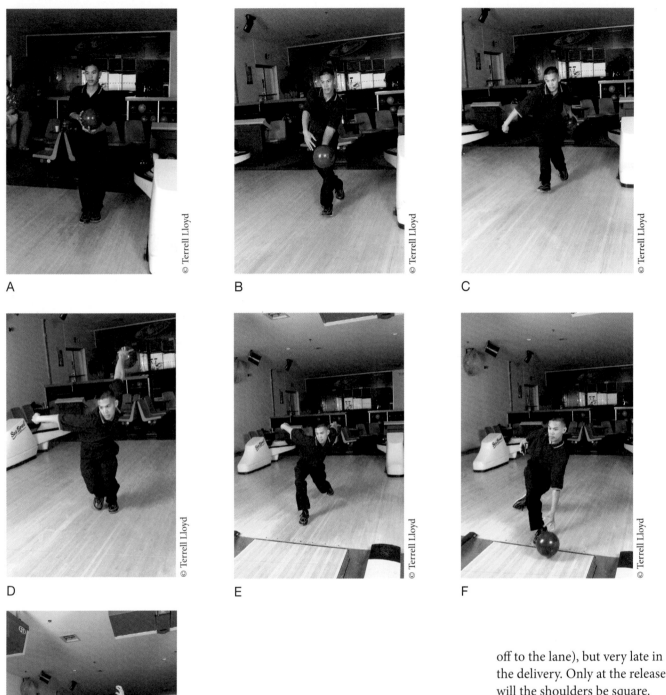

FIGURE 17.2 A—G Sequence shots of modern player's approach.

off to the lane), but very late in the delivery. Only at the release will the shoulders be square.

2. A modern player will tend to use a "coiled wrist" position (Figure 17.2). This "coiled" wrist has the wrist broken laterally left (for right handers) with the thumb facing the pins and the fingers to the left. This creates a "Frisbee-type" of release. In turn, it causes the thumb to come out of the ball very early and fast while the fingers remain

in the ball longer. All of this gives more revolutions ("revs") per minute (RPMs) that result in more effective pin carry.

3. The modern player does not emphasize the lift at the release point. In the place of lift, the advanced bowler is trying for "time differential between when the thumb exits and the fingers exit the ball." The "coiled wrist" position increases this time differential, thereby creating even greater pin reaction. Therefore, lift is becoming an obsolete term because the modern bowler seeks RPMs (revolutions per minute) instead. More RPMs can be achieved through the coiled wrist position at release.

As you can see, the modern-day bowling environment is changing in this world of technology. Although learning the basics of proper bowling technique is essential, the changing environments now found in bowling establishments and new equipment are dictating that each bowler make changes and adaptations to progress in the bowling world.

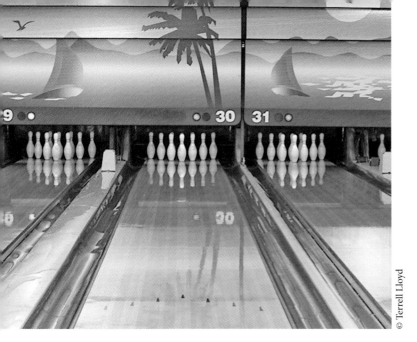
© Terrell Lloyd

18

Competitive Bowling

Philosophy of Competition

An early establishment of basic philosophy and objectives leads to success in any endeavor. Competitive bowling is no exception. The coach and each individual bowler should identify his or her own philosophy of competition and respective goals to plan a systematic course for achievement of those goals.

At the same time, however, a competitor should not lose sight of another very important objective—that of enjoyment.

The sections that follow will provide additional suggestions for goal achievement and help make your coaching responsibilities more enjoyable and successful.

Psychology of Competition

Once the technical fundamentals have been refined to successful habits, the game of bowling becomes more of a mental challenge. Almost 80 percent of one's continued success is attributable to *concentration* and one's ability to determine and adjust to the subtle variations in conditions.

The bowler must be able to *"feel"* the momentum and *"sense"* the swing of the ball, even while under great pressure. Going for the fourth or fifth strike in a row should be just the same as trying for the first one, but it seldom is. Subtle tension and pressure, not to mention mechanical variations, must be detected and neutralized.

Concentration is the name of the game. Concentration is an awareness of self in the required movement and the absence of outside thoughts. During competition, we should react almost automatically and continually readjust, relying upon the ingrained motor patterns already established. The bowler should be aware of the target and the objective, without cluttering the mind with outside distractions.

Another important element is the ability to isolate events. Take one ball at a time, not the entire frame, the game, the event, or the outcome. A series of good individual shots creates a good game and a winning performance. A good bowler can immediately leave an error behind and look to the next ball.

Many sports participants attribute their success or failure to luck, when in truth, luck is a minor factor. We must strive to minimize the effect of luck by making cool, logical adjustments. Luck will even itself out if we minimize its impact by the strength of our performance.

The bowler who can control his or her emotions and concentrate attention and energies on the task at hand will find the greatest success. A calm assurance is an effective approach to the game. Getting upset or angry does not enhance performance and will only ensure a loss of concentration and a probable series of poor shots.

Another key to the success of many bowlers, and other sports participants, is the ability to visualize the proper execution of the skill involved. The benefit of mental practice cannot be denied. Being able to visualize the perfect strike ball delivery while waiting for your turn to bowl can help your concentration and add to your effectiveness at the same time. All too many competitors make the very serious mistake of competing against someone on the other lane or the other team. A far better idea is to forget your opponents, their success, and their mistakes, and bowl against yourself. This way, you spend your time concentrating on your own game rather than defending against your opponents' game. If you are evenly matched and you are bowling against yourself while your opponents are bowling against you, chances are that 90 percent of the time you will win!

The successful bowler must also find a degree of competitive relaxation. That is to say, confidence and concentration are the tools with which to combat nervous tension and pressure attendant to competition. We need to have a confident and positive attitude toward the event to allow for maximum effectiveness.

One final note—"losers" have a real fear of failure and therefore almost always anticipate it. Winners, however, use small setbacks as stepping stones for improvement and eventual success. Losing is not to be feared, not even considered, in the winner's search for success. One of the greatest lessons in winning is to learn not to defeat yourself. To succeed, you must eliminate the fear of failure, take the game of bowling one delivery at a time, and concentrate on your own performance. Remember the winner's attitude is one of "I will," and the loser continues to say "I can't."

Mental Aspects of the Game

Once again, pick a key reminder to focus on during the approach. Avoid over thinking and the inevitable "paralysis by analysis." Trust your muscle memory so that you allow your muscles to execute what you have trained them to do. The purpose of practice is really to train the subconscious mind. When the delivery counts, allow the subconscious to function. Another way to say it is: "Trust is a must!"

- Use mental imagery, whether it be in practice or when it counts. Visualize yourself executing the approach, or any aspect of it, perfectly. Visualize the ball path on its road to a strike or a spare conversion.
- Practice mental bowling. In a comfortable, relaxed setting, bowl an entire game in your mind. Make all your approaches and results for strikes and spares a success. Mental bowling must always be positive.
- Keep thinking while bowling—in other words, pay attention to valuable information that your ball and pins could be giving you concerning the bowling environment.
- Keep an even temperament no matter what the immediate result or pinfall. Losing one's temper is

just as bad as becoming overly elated—it causes difficulties in retrieving one's concentration.

- Concentration is not the same as thinking. Thinking should happen in between deliveries, not during them. Concentration is the focusing of one's attention and trust in the subconscious muscle memory.
- When feeling tense, take one or two deep breaths before stepping up onto the approach.
- Always believe in yourself no matter the result—no one comes through with a strike all the time. Nobody's game stays great forever; it tends to go in cycles.
  1. Look for a key that enhances a performance.
  2. Find a key.
  3. Try to keep that key.
  4. Inevitably, you will lose that key, so start the process all over again.

Even in a stressful situation, or when you feel nervous, focus your attention on your form and zero in on simply rolling the ball to your target. When nerves are involved, reduce the game to its simplest elements.

Coaching Ideas

The duty of a coach is to assist the athlete or performer in achieving optimal success in the pursuit of excellence. In order to achieve this objective, a bowling coach must organize individualized practices. Each individual should be aware of the goals and objectives of each practice session for meaningful and productive practice to take place.

The following are some suggestions on how to approach the coaching of bowling and the conducting of practices:

- Remember that you are a coach/teacher and not a participant.

Your duty is to assist each of the bowlers, rather than to improve upon your own game.

- Know your bowling fundamentals and materials. Respect for you as a coach can only be obtained if the coach knows what he or she is talking about.
- Praise first and then present constructive criticism. Try to present everything in a positive manner.
- Give only one or two corrections at a time. If a coach over-instructs and gives the bowler too many things to think about at once, very little will be accomplished.
- Show enthusiasm and positivism. Both of these are contagious and will assist in fun and productive practices.
- Constant repetition enhances learning.
- Always look for the cause of the problem rather than trying to remedy the symptom.
- Individualize the practices.
- Make the other team members aware of each bowler's faults and errors. At some crucial time they may have to help each other.
- During practice, stress complete concentration and practice to eliminate poor habits. Don't allow "horseplay."
- Practice in the same type of clothing each individual will be wearing during competition.
- It is sometimes advantageous to practice in a match game situation, one against another.
- Develop ways to motivate each individual to want ultimate success.
- Work toward team rapport and team cohesiveness.
- Use visual playback methods whenever possible.
- Eliminate the fear of failure. Emphasize that a loss is merely a temporary setback. The winner's motto is: "I can" and "We will."

Suggestions on How to Adjust to Lane Conditions

Once the bowler has "read" the lane condition, or at least has a general feel for it, the following is a list of possible adjustments that could be made. The list goes from the easiest to the most difficult adjustments to make.

1. For "slow" or "dry" lanes, move the starting position to the left. Don't be afraid to move 5 or more boards. For "fast" or "wet" lanes, move the starting position to the right.

2. Move both the target and the starting position. Move the target at least one arrow and realign the starting position.

3. Change the bowling ball. For slow lanes, use a shinier, less porous bowling ball. It will skid farther down the lane. For fast lanes, use a duller, more porous bowling ball. It will grab the lane sooner.

4. Use a bowling ball with different roll and hook ability. Bowling balls can be drilled to change the arc point of the ball path, and the hooking and rolling characteristics of the ball.

5. Move your aiming point (target) further forward down the lane on a slow condition. This causes the bowler to project the ball further down the lane with greater extension. Move your aiming point closer in on a fast lane. This will aid in setting the ball down earlier and getting the ball to roll sooner.

6. The bowler could move the starting position forward or backward on the approach that, in turn, alters the release point of the bowling ball. Move back to get more roll; move forward to move up.

7. The bowler could alter the amount of speed with which the ball is delivered. Use more speed for slow lanes; less speed for fast lanes.

8. The bowler could change the hand position to increase or decrease the amount of hook. Starting with the hand further under the ball will increase hook; starting with the fingers more on the side of the ball will decrease hook.

9. The bowler could increase or decrease the amount of lift applied to the ball at the release point.

10. The bowler could alter the position of the wrist during the swing and the release. Cupping the wrist increases roll and hook; flexing it backward decreases lift.

11. The bowler could "stand taller" at the foul line (less knee bend) to create more "loft" on a slow lane condition. This would tend to increase the amount the ball skids. The bowler could also increase knee bend at the release point to release the ball earlier and cause the ball to roll sooner on an oily lane.

Obviously, adjustment possibilities 6 through 11 are more difficult to execute consistently as they may affect timing, balance, and a bowler's "normal" release. However, in a competitive scenario, they can be a valuable tool.

When reactive resin equipment is used, the bowler must remember that oil tends to "carry" or migrate down the lane quicker with use of these bowling balls. The purpose of adjusting when using reactive equipment is to ensure that the ball arrives at the same "arc" point far down the lane. Potentially, larger foot and target adjustments might need to be made; small adjustments are almost unnecessary.

With use of this equipment by more advanced bowlers, accuracy is less critical. Instead, speed adjustments are useful for getting the ball down to the correct "break point" 45 feet away. A bowler will usually find it necessary to trust selecting and aiming for a target further to the right than "normal." This is because reactive bowling balls, with their stored energy, will charge back to the pocket more strongly and sharply.

Teaching More Experienced Bowlers

Teaching and coaching experienced bowlers requires individual analysis as to the specific problem (i.e., finding the cause of the error to relieve the symptom). The teacher/coach must have the ability to distinguish between style and fundamental errors that keep a bowler from increasing pinfall. Style is the effect that our individual personalities have on our technique. An easy-going person will tend to develop a slower-tempo approach with a more "finesse" type of delivery. A more "on-the-go" person will tend to have quicker footwork and generally a more energetic delivery. Either bowler can develop skills to a high degree; the same fundamentals apply to both. Effective coaching requires working on the fundamentals and only altering a bowler's "style" when that style prevents the bowler from executing those fundamentals.

To find the errors, the bowler must be observed and analyzed from the ball side. The bowler should be observed from four different perspectives (four different locations on the approach area):

1. From directly behind the bowler's line of swing.
2. A profile view from the side at the approximate location of the second or third steps.
3. A profile view at the foul line.
4. A front view by being observed from the ball return cover or walkway beside the lane about 10 feet forward of the foul line.

The more deliveries that are observed, the easier it becomes to find the cause of the error, but at least three or four approaches should be observed before a correction is suggested.

The bowler should be observed from at least two of the above-mentioned four locations before corrections are suggested. Most helpful observation locations are from behind the line of swing and either profile view.

Most major errors can be traced back to the beginning of the approach—stance and initial movement of the ball. It is difficult to make adjustments in mid-approach for faults created in the beginning; therefore, inconsistency develops. Corrections need to be made in the right sequence:

1. Correct alignment of the bowler to the target.
2. Correct errors in the basic stance.
3. Correct errors in the initial movement of the ball in relation to the steps.
4. Make any needed corrections in swing—direction, height, wrist rotation, hand position, and so on.
5. Make any needed correction in footwork—length of steps, tempo, shuffles, knee flexion, and so on.
6. Make any needed correction in the balance line at release point— both vertical and horizontal.

7. Make any needed corrections in follow-through—height and direction.
8. Make improvements in the release of the ball—lift, rotation, wrist position, and so on.
9. Make corrections to the bowling environment—lane conditions, equipment, and so on.

Making corrections in more advanced bowling is basically learning to correct poor habits and patterns. Correcting a habit will, by necessity, feel awkward. To effect a change, a bowler must be willing to accept the feeling of awkwardness—any new motion or position tends to feel "funny" or "weird." There will not be instant success, but the bowler must be willing to practice a single correction for two to five games, after which the correction (new habit) will feel less awkward. A bowler must not expect to get a positive result (a strike) after merely one or two deliveries. Some corrections may take less practice time while others may take longer.

To correct a habit, a bowler will find it helpful to feel like he or she is "over-exaggerating" the new motion until he or she senses the difference between correct and incorrect. Once the muscles have memorized the new motion, over-exaggeration is no longer necessary (two to five games).

Focus in on a key—one thing in a bowler's approach at a time. Over-thinking creates even more problems, the main one being "paralysis by analysis" whereby the bowler loses all natural feel of the approach and armswing.

The use of a video camera is helpful in identifying errors and making corrections. It helps the bowler actually see the error, because most bowlers do not realize or really feel what they do. Nor do they visualize the appearance of their own bowling approaches.

Avoid accepting advice from anyone and everyone—it can be confusing and even contradictory. Corrections and adjustments that work for one bowler might not work, or even apply, to another bowler.

To increase one's average and skills, one must be willing to make changes in one's bowling approach and to learn about new techniques and adjustments.

How to Practice

In all sports, we equate practice with repetition of the actual game process. Bowling is no different. We say we are practicing when, in fact, we are bowling for a high score rather than for improving various elements of our game.

The following suggestions are provided in an attempt to make practice sessions more productive in contributing to improvement and refining very specific techniques:

- Don't keep score.
- Roll your second ball first, shoot for a 7 pin or a 10 pin, then roll your strike ball.
- Practice for a particular reason, such as making a correction or change.
- Concentrate on only one or two things in a given practice session.
- Over-exaggerate your corrections at first until they become natural.
- Don't be excited about strikes.
- Be happy with making a satisfactory change in your game even though there might not be an immediate result.
- It is better to practice for shorter lengths of time (30 to 60 minutes) than to do marathon practice sessions. Quality is better than quantity.
- Practice only as long as you can make a mental effort to

correct an error or learn a new adjustment—only practice with a purpose in mind. Bowling 50 games a week, for example, without a conscious effort to learn something new, will only establish poor habits.

- Deliver each practice ball as if you need it to win the game.
- Practice different angles to the pocket—for example, deliver three consecutive shots to the pocket across three different arrows.
- Vary the time of day that you practice to experience different lane conditions. Practice at different bowling centers.
- Make use of the "shadow bowling" capability of some lanes.

- Practice with a knowledgeable buddy who can correctly assist you in diagnosing your progress on one or two factors.
- Practice your concentration.
- Go to a quiet area, one with the smallest number of distractions and interruptions.
- If available, videotape or movie feedback provides an excellent resource for error analysis and correction.
- Give new techniques a chance to work. Don't expect miracles overnight.
- Remember, concentrated practice sessions can be enhanced by effective mental practice.
- Maintain your confidence. Don't give up on a new idea too soon.

Appendix A

Glossary of Terms

ABC— American Bowling Congress; a former bowling governing organization.

Alley— The 60-foot maple-pine or synthetic surface in front of the foul line on which the ball is rolled (more commonly known today as the lane).

Anchor— The last or fifth person in a team's line-up.

Angle— A combination of the direction of the delivery and the path the ball takes toward the pins.

Approach— Area behind the foul line where the bowler executes steps and delivery.

Arrows— Aiming targets embedded in the lane to help a bowler align the starting position on the approach with the ball path down the lane.

Average— Figure reached by dividing the sum of games or scores by the number of games bowled in one session or season.

Baby Split— Any split where the ball must be rolled in between, 2-7, 3-10, 4-5, 5-6, 7-8, or 9-10.

Backup Ball— A reverse hook; a ball that curves from left to right on the lane (for a right hander).

Bed Post— The 7-10 split.

Big Four— The 4-6-7-10 split.

Blind Score— Score given a team for its absent member.

Block— The application or build-up of oil in the center of the lane that, illegally, helps guide the ball to the pocket.

Boards— Individual strips of wood that make up the lane and approach.

Body English— Physical gyrations after the ball has been delivered, as if to steer the ball.

BPAA— The Bowling Proprietors Association of America; association of bowling center operators.

Break Point— The place on the lane (about 45 feet from the foul line) where the ball begins its hook.

Bridge— The distance between the finger holes.

Brooklyn Strike— A ball crossing into the 1-2 pocket resulting in a strike (right handers).

Bucket— The 2-4-5-8 and 3-5-6-9 leaves.

Channel— Accepted term for the gutter.

Cherry— To chop; to miss a pin of a 2-pin spare.

Chop— Picking a cherry.

Clean Game— A game with a mark in every frame.

Conditioner— The oil or dressing applied over the surface of the lane to prepare it for play.

Crossover— A ball going to the 1-2 pocket side for a right hander, 1-3 for a left hander.

Curve— A ball that moves to the left from the moment it is delivered. Not a hook that waits until it nears the pins before breaking to the left.

Cushion— Barrier at the rear of the pit that absorbs the pins and balls.

Dead Ball— A ball with very little action; little pin carry.

Deadwood— Pins left down on the pin deck after the first ball of a frame.

Decks (Pin Decks)— The area of the lane where the pins are placed.

Double— Two consecutive strikes.

Double Pinochle— The 4-6-7-10 set-up.

Dutch 200— A 200 game scored by rolling alternate frames of spares and strikes.

Error— A miss.

Fast— Lanes that hold down the hook; sometimes referred to as "oily" or "slick." Today these lanes are more accurately referred to as "holding."

Flip— Extreme delay in the motion of ball; right-to-left association with reactive resin bowling balls.

Foul— The act of going beyond the foul line as you deliver the ball.

Frame— One-tenth of a game.

Full Hit— A ball that hits squarely on the head pin. Used to describe any ball that hits the target squarely or dead center.

Full Roller— A hook type of release in which the thumb rotates 10 to 11 o'clock and fingers lift through the ball for a right hander.

Goal Posts— The 7-10 split.

Grave Yard— The toughest lanes on which to produce good scores.

Gutter— Channel on each side of the bowling lane.

Handicap— Adjustment in score totals between individuals or teams to equalize competition.

Head Pin — The number 1 pin.

Heads — The first 15 to 17 feet of the lane onto which the ball is released.

High Hit, Heavy Hit — A strike ball that comes into the head pin more than the 3 pin of the 1-3 pocket.

Hook — A ball that breaks from right to left well after release (for right handers).

House Ball — A ball provided by the bowling center for customer use.

Kickback — Side partitions between lanes at the pit end.

King Pin — The 5 pin.

Lane — Sixty-foot maple-pine or synthetic surface in front of the foul line on which the ball is rolled; also called an alley.

Leadoff — The first person on a team.

League — An organized group of teams competing on a regular, formal basis under a specific code of rules and regulations.

Leave — The pins left standing after the first ball has been rolled.

Lift — Giving the ball an upward motion with the fingers at the point of release.

Light Hit, Thin Hit — Strike ball that fails to come up into the 1-3 pocket; hits more on the 3 pin than the head pin.

Line — The path of the ball from release point to the pocket.

Locator Dots — The 3 rows of dots on the approach.

Lofting — Throwing the ball out on the lane well beyond the foul line so it drops from a height.

Mark — A strike or a spare.

Miss, Error, Blow — Ball not making contact with any pins standing.

Mixer — A good working ball that produces lively action among the pins.

NBC — The former National Bowling Council; bowling industry promotion and service organization.

Oil — The substance used to coat or dress the lanes.

Open Frame — A frame without a strike or spare.

PBA — Professional Bowler's Association; organization of male professional bowlers.

Perfect Game — A 300 game, consisting of 12 strikes in one game.

Perfect Strike — A ball that hits the pins squarely in the pocket (between the 1 and 3 pins) and clears the deck of all pins.

Picket Fence — The 1-2-4-7 or 1-3-6-10.

Pinspotter, Pinsetter — Automatic machine that picks up and sets the pins for the bowler.

Pit — Area at the end of the lane into which the pins fall.

Pitch — The angle in relation to the center of the ball at which the thumb and finger holes of a ball are drilled.

Pocket — The areas between the 1 and 3 pins (for right handers); the strike zone.

Powerhouse — A very strong hooking ball that seems to tear the pins apart.

Pumpkin — The opposite of powerhouse.

Pushaway — The outward, downward thrust of the ball that puts the ball into motion.

Reactive Resin Ball — Bowling ball with tacky surface created by a polymer added to urethane that provides more grip of the ball to the lane.

Scratch — Use of actual scores and averages in individual or team competition; non-handicap bowling.

Semi-Roller — A hook type of release in which the thumb rotates counter-clockwise (11 to 10 o'clock) and the finger lift throws the ball (right handed).

Sleeper — A hidden pin; the 8 pin in the 2-8 setup.

Slow Lane — Double meaning term used in describing a lane that either resists a hook or assists it. Varies with geographical areas.

Sour Apple — The 5-7-10 split.

Span — The distance between the thumb and finger holes.

Spare — Knocking down all 10 pins in one frame with two rolls of the ball.

Spinner — A method of release that imparts an excessive counter-clockwise rotation of the thumb (11 to 7 o'clock) for right handers.

Split — Two or more pins left standing after the first roll with a pin down immediately between or ahead of them (providing the 1 pin is down also).

Spot — A target guide on the lane used to aid the bowler in directing the ball; also term used to designate the handicap given another bowler or team.

Strike — Knock down all the pins with the first roll of the ball in a frame.

Strike Out — Three consecutive strikes in the 10th frame.

Sweep — The metal mechanism that cleans the pin deck after each delivery of the ball.

Tap — An apparently perfect strike hit that leaves the 8 pin standing.

Target Arrow — Aiming device located on the lane approximately 15 feet in front of the foul line. Also called range finder or mark.

Triple — Three strikes in succession. Also called a turkey.

Turkey — Three strikes in a row.

USBC — United States Bowling Congress; the governing organization of bowling.

USBC — Youth — The division of USBC governing youth activities in the sport.

Washout — The 1-2-10 or the 1-2-4-10 spares (right handers).

WIBC — Women's International Bowling Congress; a former organization of women bowlers.

Working Ball — Ball that moves with good rolling action; see Mixer.

Appendix B

Bowler's Analysis Chart
(Former National Bowling Council)

NAME _____ LEFT HANDED ❏   RIGHT HANDED ❏

GRIP: CONVENTIONAL ❏   FINGERTIP ❏   SEMI-FINGERTIP ❏   OTHER ❏

SPECS: WEIGHT _____   TOP ❏   SIDE ❏   FINGER ❏

TRACK: FULL ROLLER ❏   SEMI-ROLLER ❏   SPINNER ❏   OTHER ❏

STANCE COMMENTS

FEET: STRAIGHT TO INTENDED LINE   YES ❏   NO ❏

CLOSE ❏   FAIRLY CLOSE ❏   APART ❏   TOES TOGETHER ❏

LEFT FOOT AHEAD ❏   RIGHT FOOT AHEAD ❏

WEIGHT DISTRIBUTION:

MOSTLY RIGHT ❏   MOSTLY LEFT ❏   EVENLY DISTRIBUTED ❏

KNEES: BOTH BENT ❏   RIGHT BENT ❏   LEFT BENT ❏   STRAIGHT ❏

RELATIVE HEIGHT OF BALL:

CHEST HIGH ❏   WAIST HIGH ❏   KNEE HIGH ❏

ALIGNMENT OF BALL:

RIGHT OF SHOULDER ❏   IN LINE WITH SHOULDER ❏

AT CENTER LINE ❏   BETWEEN SHOULDER AND CENTER LINE ❏

WEIGHT OF BALL:

RIGHT HAND ❏   LEFT HAND ❏   DISTRIBUTED BETWEEN BOTH HANDS ❏

ELBOW: TUCKED INTO HIP ❏   AWAY FROM HIP ❏

WRIST: STRAIGHT ❏   FAIRLY STRAIGHT ❏   BENT ❏

THUMB POSITION: RELATIVE POSITION ON CLOCK _____

APPROACH
COMMENTS

NUMBER OF STEPS _____

LENGTH OF STEPS: LONG ❏ MODERATE ❏ SHORT ❏
TEMPO: FAST ❏ MODERATE ❏ SLOW ❏

HEEL-TOE ❏ SHUFFLE ❏
STRAIGHT ❏ DRIFT RIGHT ❏
DRIFT LEFT ❏

ARMSWING: PARALLEL ❏ OUTSIDE-IN ❏ INSIDE-OUT ❏
LOOP ❏ BENT ELBOW ❏

RIGHT ANGLES TO INTENDED LINE:
SHOULDERS   HIPS

RIGHT ❏   RIGHT ❏
FACING   FACING
LEFT ❏   LEFT ❏

BACKSWING: BELOW WAIST ❏ WAIST HIGH ❏
AT SHOULDER LEVEL ❏ ABOVE SHOULDER LEVEL ❏
WRIST: FIRM ❏ BENT BACK ❏ CUPPED ❏
BALANCE LINE: GOOD KNEE BEND ❏ TOO MUCH ❏ NOT ENOUGH ❏

RELEASE
COMMENTS

PALM: DOWN ❏ LEFT ❏ UP ❏ RIGHT ❏

WRIST: FIRM ❏ SAGGED ❏ ROTATES: LEFT ❏ RIGHT ❏

FINGERS: FIRM ❏ CLOSED ❏ OPEN ❏

LIFT: SMOOTH ❏ CRISP ❏ WEAK ❏

OUTSIDE FINGERS: BOTH CLOSE ❏ BOTH SPREAD ❏ INDEX FINGER
SPREAD ❏ LITTLE FINGER SPREAD ❏ LITTLE FINGER TUCKED
UNDER ❏

FOLLOW-THROUGH
COMMENTS

DIRECTION RELATIVE TO TARGET:
IN LINE ❏ RIGHT OF TARGET ❏ LEFT OF TARGET ❏ HEIGHT:
WAIST ❏ SHOULDER ❏ OVERHEAD ❏ INCONSISTENT ❏

BALL ROLL
COMMENTS

ACTION: STRAIGHT ❏ HOOK ❏ CURVE ❏ BACK-UP ❏
NUMBER OF BOARDS _____
HITTING POWER: STRONG ❏ WEAK ❏ NORMAL ❏

METHOD OF AIMING
COMMENTS   SPOT: FOUL LINE ❏   LINE

                                     DOTS   ❏   PIN ❏   SHADOW ❏   OR ❏

                                     ARROWS   ❏   AREA

SPARE SHOOTING
COMMENTS

              SPOT BOWLER: SPARE TO LEFT

                  USES STRIKE TARGET—MOVES RIGHT ❏
                  FOOT PLACEMENT SAME—TARGET MOVED ❏
                  COMBINATION ❏

              SPOT BOWLER: SPARE TO RIGHT

                  USES THIRD ARROW—MOVES FEET LEFT ❏
                  FOOT PLACEMENT SAME—TARGET MOVED ❏
                  COMBINATION ❏

COMMENTS: 1st ANALYSIS	2nd ANALYSIS	3rd ANALYSIS	4th ANALYSIS

Credits

This page constitutes an extension of the copyright page. We have made every effort to trace the ownership of all copyrighted material and to secure permission from copyright holders. In the event of any question arising as to the use of any material, we will be pleased to make the necessary corrections in future printings. Thanks are due to the following authors, publishers, and agents for permission to use the material indicated.

Chapter One
p. 5: © Terrell Lloyd; p. 7: Courtesy of former NBC; p. 8: Courtesy of former NBC; pp. 9, 10, left top, top center: © Terrell Lloyd; p. 11, bottom left: © Eric Risberg; p. 11, top right, bottom left, bottom right: © Terrell Lloyd; p. 11, top left: © Eric Risberg;

Chapter Two
pp. 13, 14: © Eric Risberg; pp. 15, 17, 20, 22: © Terrell Lloyd; p. 23, 24: © Eric Risberg; p. 22, left: © Terrell Lloyd

Chapter Three
p. 27, top left: © Terrell Lloyd; p. 27: © Eric Risberg; p. 28 top left, center:

© Eric Risberg; p. 30: right top, 29, 30, 31: © Terrell Lloyd; pp. 32, 34, bottom, top left, top right: © Eric Risberg; pp. 34, 35, 36, 37, 38, 40, 42, 43: © Terrell Lloyd

Chapter Four
pp. 45, 46, 47, 50, 51: © Terrell Lloyd

Chapter Five
pp. 53, 56, 57, 59, 60, 62: © Terrell Lloyd

Chapter Six
pp. 66, 67: Courtesy of former NBC

Chapter Seven
pp. 73, 74: © Terrell Lloyd; pp. 76, 77, 78, 79, 80, 81, 82, 83: © Eric Risberg

Chapter Eight
p. 87: © Terrell Lloyd

Chapter Nine
p. 93: Courtesy of the United States Bowling Congress

Chapter Ten
pp. 99, 100, 101, 102, 103: © Eric Risberg;

Chapter Eleven
p. 107: © Mark E. Gibson/Documentary/ CORBIS; pp. 111, 112, 113

Chapter Twelve
pp. 119, 121, 122, 123, 125: © Terrell Lloyd

Chapter Thirteen
pp. 127, 129, top left: © Terrell Lloyd; p. 129: © Eric Risberg; pp. 134, 135, 138: © Terrell Lloyd; p. 138, bottom: © Eric Risberg

Chapter Fourteen
p. 139: © Eric Risberg; p. 140, 141: © Terrell Lloyd; pp. 142, 143: © Eric Risberg

Chapter Fifteen
pp. 145, 146: Courtesy of former NBC

Chapter Sixteen
p. 149: © Terrell Lloyd; pp. 150, 151: Courtesy of former NBC

Chapter Seventeen
pp. 153, 155, 156, : © Terrell Lloyd

Chapter Eighteen
p. 159: © Terrell Lloyd

Index